CANARIES IN THE COAL MINE

A Journey of Discovery

ELAINE MARIE GRAHAM

BALBOA.
PRESS

A DIVISION OF HAY HOUSE

The Author Credits this work to Holistic Physicians Everywhere

Balboa Press books may be ordered through booksellers or by contacting:

Balboa Press
A Division of Hay House
1663 Liberty Drive
Bloomington, IN 47403
www.balboapress.com
1-(877) 407-4847

ISBN: 978-1-4525-4610-0 (sc)
ISBN: 978-1-4525-4611-7 (e)

Because of the dynamic nature of the Internet, any web addresses or links contained in this book may have changed since publication and may no longer be valid. The views expressed in this work are solely those of the author and do not necessarily reflect the views of the publisher, and the publisher hereby disclaims any responsibility for them.

The author of this book does not dispense medical advice or prescribe the use of any technique as a form of treatment for physical, emotional, or medical problems without the advice of a physician, either directly or indirectly. The intent of the author is only to offer information of a general nature to help you in your quest for emotional and spiritual well-being. In the event you use any of the information in this book for yourself, which is your constitutional right, the author and the publisher assume no responsibility for your actions.

Any people depicted in stock imagery provided by Thinkstock are models, and such images are being used for illustrative purposes only. Certain stock imagery © Thinkstock.

Printed in the United States of America

Balboa Press rev. date: 2/25/2012

DEDICATION

I dedicate this book to all who have been diagnosed with chronic fatigue/ fibromyalgia or any auto-immune disease.

To those who have given up their fight after years of suffering or shear exhaustion I send my love.

To future generations who will be dealing with this I hope to shed some much needed light on the subject in hopes that they will have the research and the knowledge to know what to do to turn their health around and have a productive and peaceful life before too much damage is done.

In Greek my name means "Torch bright light."

In Arthurian history legend Elaine was the daughter of Paellas the lover of Sir Lancelot.

In English the source of the name Elaine is Helen an English name meaning "sun ray."

May I bring a ray of sun to all who pass this way. I send you my love.

Psalms 34:21 Evil shall slay the wicked and they that hate the righteous shall be desolate.

CONTENTS

FOREWORD

Elaine has extensively studied chronic fatigue and fibromyalgia for the past 17 years. She decided to write this book about the pain and anguish involved with these disorders. There is a possible significant method we have been undergoing that has really made a change in both of our health issues discussed above.

With amazing insights into all aspects of chronic fatigue and fibromyalgia she wanted to share this information with people who desperately need the information. This is a book written from both our experiences. It has been a long journey as Elaine has had CFS/Fibromyalgia for about 17 years and I have had chronic fatigue for the past 65 years, so she is delivering our personal life experiences in dealing with and trying to overcome these disorders. Her wish is to share much of the research she has been privileged to come across which can make a significant difference in issues people are dealing with weather it is CF/FM or any auto-immune condition.

Elaine nor I are medical doctors but sometimes experience is a much better teacher than a textbook and so she brings our experiences to her book. Be prepared for an interesting journey through this complex area of health issues and hopefully you will find answers you are seeking and more importantly Elaine hopes it helps to alleviate a lot of people's pain and suffering from CFS/fibromyalgia.

Kent

Without the love and care of an understanding spouse these conditions can easily overcome someone dealing with them if they are alone. I give thanks for having a spouse that has had knowledge himself about dealing with chronic fatigue.

Elaine Marie Graham

PREFACE

I don't think anyone can imagine how scary it can be when given a diagnosis that is considered a "somato" (all in your head) form of illness; especially when you are in excruciating unrelenting pain. No one can know by looking at another human being how much pain they might be in. Fibromyalgia and chronic fatigue have been referred to as the invisible illness because you can't comprehend what is going on when it involves the immune, neurological and endocrine systems. I'm sure many children with autism may be in pain as well. I find this disturbing since children do not have the ability to tell you what they are feeling when they can't speak.

With all the research and knowledge that has been published in the last two decades about these disorders, I find it disturbing that more doctors have not been educated about them.

After going to general medical physicians and having my condition made worse by their advice, I decided to study as much as I could about how the body works and read everything I could get my hands on about the conditions of FM/CF. It has been a constant quest for knowledge about these topics. Unfortunately even the well meaning physicians who are trying to get into integrative medicine don't always have all the answers. Sometimes even though they mean well they might not have all the knowledge they need to make a proper treatment protocol. This can result in worsening the problem.

I can't think of a problem that might create more stress and emotional anguish other than being diagnosed with cancer. I confess that I have had times, and I know others have as well, wished that I could be released from this world and the suffering in it. Something has pushed me to cling on in hopes of finding the answers. I don't know what that push in me is if it is stubbornness or my hope of finding the answers so that others might not have to endure the pain and anguish I have had to deal with. I did make a promise to God if I found the answers; I would share them with as many people as possible.

I have had too many years of struggling with medical bills and not seeing the progress I hoped to see. Dr. Cheney said, "these people are loaded with all kinds of chemicals and heavy metals and they have to be detoxed to get well."

It is however almost impossible to get rid of metals when your liver detox pathways are impaired and you have a block in the methylation pathways. I have learned that this is key when you're dealing with detoxing metals. The most important thing you can do for your healing is to raise the glutathione production so toxins can be cleared from the system and hopefully the detox pathways will be restored. You also need to work on your nutritional status.

My condition became much worse when they tried to chelate heavy metals. I was nutritionally deficient in B-12, B-6 and zink. My liver detox pathways were also not working well. This caused a worsening of my condition and caused a number of auto-immune symptoms.

There is a brilliant physician and researcher who have patented a product that raises your glutathione levels by feeding the cells what they need to make their own glutathione. I believe this will be key to any health challenge.

Since my husband has been on this product, he has seen such a surge in his energy, it is hard to believe. He is now able to exercise without needing a nap and taking two days to recover. He now can exercise and still have energy through the rest of the day. It no longer takes him two days to recover. He is so excited, he can't wait to share this product with his physician. In fact we were told that many physicians are using this remarkable product in their medical practices and one physician gave up his practice to travel about and give seminars on this remarkable product and the company that produces it.

We think the knowledge of this product and what it can do to improve anyone's health will change the face of healthcare.

I am also having a sense of better health, however my challenges are a little greater due to years of carrying around toxic metals and the injuries I sustained. My hope is the longer I am on this product, the better my health will become. We can't say enough about this because we have spent a fortune and tried so many different therapies to try and restore our health. We now want to share the knowledge we have gained through our experiences with you the readers.

FIBROMYALGIA/CHRONIC FATIGUE MY STORY

In the early 90's those who developed chronic fatigue/ fibromyalgia were referred to as canaries in the coal mine. I don't know who started this saying, but as it turns out it is very clear that we are in the throws of a great awakening here on planet earth.

Researchers are finding that many of the issues in autism are also present in fibromyalgia/chronic fatigue. These issues are digestive problems, low glutathione, cognitive problems, food intolerances, heavy metals, imbalance in neurotransmitters, poor methylation of toxins etc. Many feel very strongly there is of course a connection to toxin exposures and the development of these conditions. I feel there is no longer any doubt that these connections have been proven.

I learned through research that coal miners would carry cages of small canaries into the coal mines to worn them when there were toxic gases that might be in the area they were working. When a canary fell off its perch, they knew they had to get out of the coal mine fast or they also might fall prey to the toxic gases that were present.

I developed these conditions of chronic fatigue/ fibromyalgia after having a shoulder injury at work which lead into a very frozen shoulder. This would require three hours of surgery and months of torturous physical therapy to restore movement and function to the shoulder joint.

I wouldn't learn until much later that I was dealing with exposures to many heavy metals.

The movement of the shoulder wasn't much better after the surgery. It took three hours to free up some of the adhesions that by this time had to be cut out. The doctor also shaved some bone so that it would make some space in case of more swelling. There isn't any worse pain than bone that has been cut on or scraped. This resulted in constant burning pain which would keep me from getting a good nights sleep for a couple of weeks.

Doing anything around the house such as dishes or running a sweeper created more pain and inflammation and made the physical therapy sessions much harder to tolerate. My husband had to step in an do the things I normally would do around the house. If I had been allowed therapy right away; it might have prevented the surgery. Because I first had a chiropractor ask for therapy, they would not approve it. By the time I got into therapy the shoulder was so frozen I couldn't even comb my hair and there was no way to reverse the damage that had been done other than surgery and physical therapy.

If you can imagine having adhesions which hold the tissues together being torn in order to get movement back into the shoulder then you might be able to comprehend what I mean when I say torturous physical therapy. Each time I went to therapy they had to stress the adhesions which causes tearing of the tissues. I don't think there is any physical therapy that could cause more pain with the exception of a frozen knee. I wouldn't wish this problem on my worst enemy. I would suggest to anyone dealing with a frozen shoulder they look at my article on tests you should have for fibromyalgia. (You'll find this at the end of this book.) They obviously have a lot of inflammation in their body. Of course injury can also cause inflammation.

Being a very determined individual, I decided to do whatever it might take to get the movement and function back which I previously had. They also had to free the scapula which was still frozen when I came out of surgery. This was especially painful. One therapist held the scapula in will the other one forced the shoulder joint to move! They wanted to do more that day but the pain was too great. I know that they were frustrated that my progress had been so slow because they said they were afraid the doctor would think they hadn't been doing anything. I can now only imagine that the stress hormones I was producing were tearing up my intestinal tract and searing my tissues. This is what happens when you produce a lot of cortisol which is the stress hormone produced by the adrenals. Too much production becomes toxic to the body and can also lead to a metabolic wasting syndrome.

I went back to work gradually just working 3-4 hour days. I really was determined to get my full function back. I also had a son in college so it wasn't a good time for me to be disabled. He obviously needed my help. This of course put a lot of stress on me at that time.

When I was re-injured due to straining the neck and shoulders, I had to go back off work. I was without income for around 8 mo. because the doctor's office failed to properly process the paperwork. When I expressed my concern to the doctor, he got my disability payments started right away.

One thing I never wanted to be was disabled. My father developed type I diabetes in his mid thirties. I saw what being disabled does to a person. It narrows your life down to just the bare necessities and many times you might not have the money to deal with extra things that come up in life. I watched him deteriorate to the point where his life was spent mostly in his chair. He was however very interested in world events and always watched the news. My father taught me to be an independent thinker. He always said never believe everything you read, hear or see; try to get the full picture so you know what is going on.

My father was a very wise man. He tried to eat mostly organic food and raised some of his own beef. Of course he didn't use steroids or hormones with his animals. I remember some roast he gave me and it tasted so different from the store bought beef. It was much more flavorful. Of course it was grass feed. He read Prevention Magazine and tried to learn all he could about maintaining his Type I diabetes from a holistic viewpoint. My father was a veteran and served in the Philippines. I often wondered if he could have picked up something in the service that lead to his diabetes. I never thought about the mercury in the vaccines; but recently I read an opinion that mercury could indeed cause the immune system to attack the pancreas. This is very scary to me. None of his 6 siblings ever developed diabetes. I think we attribute too many things to genes.

I don't doubt that toxins could cause the immune system to attack an organ they have connected this to thyroid disease as well as diabetes. They now know chemical and metal toxins can cause antibodies to be produced by the immune system. I have also read that some drugs can affect the pancreas and this may be why I wasn't producing enough amylase to break down carbs after my injury. It has been stated that high pyrovates in the blood is one of the metabolic imbalances in fibromyalgia. (See article on metabolic origin later in this book.)

My father had open heart surgery when he was in his late 60's. There were 5 doctors standing by because of his fragile condition. There were several people having surgery that day, but the doctors were amazed that he came through the surgery better than all the other patients. He had his surgery in a V.A. Hospital. I was very impressed with his care, the nurses and doctors were great!

I'm sure my father's years of taking anti-oxidants and supplements had a lot to do with the fact that he came through this so well. I remember seeing a program that had a nurse who was only maybe in her forties and she had double amputations. You could see she was wasting away and she was very distraught over her condition. She said, "I just didn't take care of myself."

My father never had any body parts amputated but he did have failing eyesight before he passed. He was 76 when he passed. We were all amazed at how long he lived and how well he did considering his uncontrollable blood sugars. I'm sure his dedication to learning all he could about the natural approach to health is what kept him going and from succumbing to amputations.

SUBSEQUENT INJURY DUE TO WEAKENED MUSCLES

Unfortunately I would suffer another injury after returning to work because the muscles never regained the strength they should have had. The fact that they changed the work station which put more strain on the neck and shoulders two weeks before I would be re-injured did not help. I did report that I didn't feel the station was very ergonomic due to this change, but nothing was done about changing the work station. This is what is referred to in worker's comp. as failure to accommodate. My co-worker who hadn't had an injury was also complaining about the stress on her shoulders from the additional strain of lifting against the weight of the tubs we were required to lift.

I didn't realize I had lost all the natural curve of the neck, but the last day I worked I had blurry vision and a nagging headache. When I reported to the nurse, my blood pressure was quite high which wasn't normal for me at that time. The loss of curvature of the neck was later diagnosed as radiculopathy. Interestingly, when I got my records from my insurance provider they claimed I didn't have radiculopathy or the neurological symptoms that you have with fibromyalgia. I now know you need to ask for reports that are in the insurance records to be sure you know what is in them. Long term disability insurers have had many class action lawsuits against them. I just read that one in particular is still denying claims they were ordered to honor. This was on Lawyers and Settlements web site. They are finding that insurer is still not paying claims they were ordered to pay. Claimants should not have to deal with all this stress. I get periodic updates from Lawyers and Settlements on the latest lawsuits they are pursuing, and some of the cases of antibiotic reactions are quite scary. It is interesting to follow the latest suits against drugs etc. This is my go to website for the latest information on drug side affects.

Anyone who has suffered with true fibromyalgia knows that you get brain fog and this interferes with memory, concentration and processing of thoughts! I have also had times when I can't pull a word from my memory or am asked a question only to think of something I should have said much later. I have a friend who says sometimes it is like someone pulled a plug in your brain and you just lose your train of thought. I have observed her doing this and experienced it myself at times.

No doubt my headache and blurry vision were the result of the stress in the neck from bending the neck forward while putting a strain on the muscles and nerves. My orthopedic surgeon diagnosed me as having a chronic neck strain. I have been told I should have sued him but there is no way he could have known that I would develop these problems while doing the lifting he told me to continue to do. I had complained to him of shoulder pain and pain where the bicept tendon had to be trimmed. He said, "just keep doing what your doing and your shoulder will get stronger." Under normal circumstances I should have gotten back full function. He also said he was surprised my shoulder was as good as it was; he didn't think I would ever be that good! The worker's comp physician they sent me to said he had never seen a shoulder that bad and didn't know what work I could do with my shoulder condition. My scapula was still partially frozen at this point. Of course he didn't put what he told me into the record.

I have some narrowing of a disc in the mid neck region and some arthritis no doubt due to injury. I would learn much later that I had been exposed to many toxic metals through a job I had done. Metals like lead and antimony are known to cause weakness in the joints and muscles.

When you injure a joint the body dumps calcium there to try and deal with the problem, but this can lead to pain and arthritis much later.

I had a large piece of calcium in the bursa of the shoulder after injuring it. I believe without chelation therapy I might not have regained movement because I believe the calcium was causing a lot of restriction. I had a few chelation treatments for this and all of this calcium was dissolved.

The doctor said he had never seen anything like that. This physician also did chelation for metals. I don't know why he didn't look for metals at this time. He reported to me that he thought the leaky gut syndrome was the cause of the fibromyalgia/chronic fatigue syndrome I developed after the injury.

CHEMICAL EXPOSURES CAUSE MUSCLE WEAKNESS

My orthopedic surgeon could also not have known that toxins I had been exposed to could be driving some of the inflammation I was experiencing. My insurer said my treating physician agreed that I could return to work. He said I might try it if they could find something where I could use arm and hand splints which would also support the shoulders. Actually this was the suggestion from UNUM Disability Insurance carrier. They wrote him a letter with this request. He laughed when he told me about it and said "they won't find a job like that." My condition continued to deteriorate. He then said I would never be able to return to my former work and that I was totally and permanently disabled from all gainful employeement. The insurer never told me this nor did my worker's comp attorney. I learned this much later when I asked for my records from the insurance company. This was only the beginning of my life's challenges. They terminated my policy at the two year own occupation limit. The language of the policy stated that I would receive payment for as long as my physician found me to be disabled. This language was changed some time after I became disabled. I ask the company for the information on when this changed but never received a reply to this question.

My chronic neck strain was a flow through injury but when I was diagnosed with fibromyalgia my employer said it was "something medical" and placed me on long term disability. They denied everything under worker's comp. It is ironic that later when I learned I had been exposed to many neuro-toxins from a lead soldering job and other exposures like welding on small welding machines. The empolyer then said I asked for coverage for the fibromyalgia under workers comp before I signed off the shoulder injury. They presented a form in court that the lawyer had submitted but it did not contain my signature and I don't remember him ever telling me he was submitting this form. In fact when I signed off the shoulder injury because they wouldn't give me anything more than a partial permanent disability; I was told by the attorney that the chronic fatigue and fibromyalgia had nothing to do with the worker's comp case and should not interfere with collecting on that policy. The Department of Labor now says this is a worker's comp claim.

I believe anyone dealing with worker's comp or a long term disability insurance company should be given all correspondence from their physician. This would stop some of the injustice that has been going on in our courts and with long term disability insurance companies. They should also not be able to rule on a case solely on the statement of a physician they hire to examine you only once. These physicians are not familiar with your case and have never treated you. We obviously need reform in the worker's comp system and the long term disability insurance companies. Ironically our representatives in congress never have to deal with either of these issues they have their own private insurance. If they did have to deal with these things, I believe the concerns of policy holders would be addressed.

Worker's rights have been destroyed for too long. The government should be protecting these rights. Someone who has been disabled because of a company's willful act of ignoring a material safety data sheet or hazard violation, should not have to sue to get their rights honored. The states should be going after these safety violators and harassers not the injured person. There was a petition on "We The People" to this affect just recently. I find it curious labor law petitions are not there very long and seem to just disappear. If you watched the Republican debates, you may have picked up on the fact that politicians are themselves talking about the failure of the worker's comp system and the judicial system. One presidential hopeful stated that the president has the duty and the right to overturn any judge's decision that is not appropriate. They also stated that lawyers are acting like judges by deciding what the law should be and proceeding accordingly instead of following the laws already on the books.

We need oversight of our courts. They should have to provide a clerk to take notes of any hearing. Anyone who has had a lawyer who failed to fairly represent them should have a lawyer appointed by the state who is paid for by the workers of the state. This could be taken out of the workers comp administration funds. Instead of boards who represent the state, we need lawyers who represent the people. This would bring back justice to the system. Of course corporations have all the lawyers they need because they have the money to pay for them. Injured worker's are losing their rights because lawyers are failing to properly represent them.

The Supreme Court rule in Ohio on toxic tort issues states that the employee's time to sue does not start to run until you learn that something your employer did exposed you to a toxic substance. The ruling came from Justice Frances E. Sweeney. He states, "To deny an employee the right to file an action before he or she discovers that the injury was caused by the employer's wrongful conduct is to deny the employee the right to bring any claim at all." "By applying the discovery rule as we do, we take away the advantage of employers who conceal harmful information until it is too late for their employees to use it." I don't know the laws for other states but they should be similar.

The case this was sited from is Norgard v. Brush Wellman, Inc., Lawyers Weekly No. 100-157-02. Mr. Norgard had symptoms of beryllium exposure for 15 years before he learned that his employer had done something that exposed him to this toxic substance. Obviously this rule was ignored when my lawyers allowed my case to proceed to civil court. Any judge who ignores the Supreme Court rule of laws of any state should be removed from the bench as unfit to serve his duties.

I have had tort lawyers tell me they will not take a tort case any longer in Ohio because they know they can't win in that state. They also said they need people like me to make a lot of noise about what is going on to help them get reform in the system. There is something wrong with the system that does not police itself. There is something wrong with the judicial system obviously. The problem as I see it is favoritism. I was told by the first worker's comp lawyer that it wasn't politically correct to be on the side of the injured worker.

The welding rod exposure cases in Cuyahoga County keep being denied. The only case that has been allowed was due to the injured person developing Parkinson's from manganese poisoning. You can read about these cases by doing a search on welding rod exposures in Cuyahoga County, Cleveland, Ohio.

Ironically when Governor Strickland was in office he said that we need a one stop shop in Ohio for heavy metal exposures. Since he understood the seriousness of this issue, I don't understand how he allowed these cases to keep being denied and bounced around in the court system. When I wrote him, he said he didn't have jurisdiction over these issues that I should write the attorney general's office. I learned that my lawyer had been appointed by him to serve on the worker's comp board. He actually was receiving a salary from them. I don't think any lawyer who is representing himself as an injured worker's lawyer should be placed in a position to work for the state. When I complained to the Supreme Court they questioned him on this. He said he didn't have anything to do with decisions made on cases. I would like to know just what role he did play. He obviously let my case go to court without the proper information in the hearing reports. I never claimed I got the exposure just from fumes. I said we weren't given gloves and were never given the material safety data sheet. I also said several of the employees including myself were asked to scrape splattered soldering material from parts for two days. OSHA has guidelines that state anyone who is doing such a process should check with HPO for directions on safety measures before proceeding to do this kind of work. This is due to the fact that particles can become airborne and you might inhale them. We were not given any safety precautions that might prevent this.

I now know the drugs, exposures to chemicals and metals along with the trauma of the shoulder injury no doubt lead to my conditions of chronic fatigue/fibromyalgia, digestive disturbances and the long list associated with these conditions. You can carry metals for years and only become reactive when you develop leaky gut syndrome. You may however have nutrient deficiencies and this is their toxic affect. This may present itself as a weakened immune system, endocrine problems, food intolerances, depression, personality changes and a host of other problems, along with creating auto-immune reactions within the immune system. Latent effects can cause renal failure and encephalopathy of the brain. It is malpractice when doctors fail to check for these conditions. Patients have been wrongly diagnosed for years.

The employer video taped me picking up small pine cones to prove that I could work. My physician said, "do not take this personally, they do it to everyone." I had to take pain pills and muscle relaxers after doing this small amount of activity. I would also have to have steroid injections into the muscles of my back from just lifting something which was no more than 5 lbs. I just turned wrong when I bent over and I could hardly straighten back up. I couldn't even turn over in bed because of the severe pain that would shoot through the muscles up into the neck. I had to have steroid injections into the muscles, these injections were extremely painful. The doctor stated, "I'm proud of you, you took that like a real woman, I have seen grown men fall on the flour and cry when they have had these injections."

ADAAA DISABILITY RULES

There was a case which I think further explains what is considered a disabling condition this is clearly spelled out in the Americans with Disabilities Act. You don't have to have a condition that is so totally limiting or excludes any life activities. One of the stated purposes of the ADAAA is to reject the standards of "substantially limits" and "major life activities" expressed in one case concerning an employee of Toyota. It wasn't intended to make the level of disability so high that it "creates an inappropriately high level of limitation necessary to obtain coverage under the ADA." I found this information on Employment Law from the library.

I find it disturbing when I see infomercials of people being filmed working that are on worker's comp. They may have had no choice but to try and work due to the fact that it can take an inordinate amount of time to even get a hearing for worker's comp in Ohio and I'm sure it isn't any better anywhere else!

People keep telling me Indiana is worse than Ohio when it comes to worker's comp but I did find a case in the newspaper where the lady was given social security disability after a two year battle with the system. She was dealing with fibromyalgia. This is a far cry from what I had to deal with; I was fighting them for 8 years. I have read some of the problems people in Ca. have encountered with this program. Many working people can't afford to be without a paycheck for any length of time. Of course they didn't recognize fibromyalgia as a disabling condition when I became disabled by it, they did however have quidelines for chronic fatigue syndrome which they ignored in my case.

To ensure that the ADA is interpreted correctly, the EEOC was directed to change its interpretation of "substantially limits a major life activity" to something less restrictive. It now states that a major life activity includes major bodily functions, such as the proper functioning of the immune system and normal cell growth.

They now know that there are disturbances in the immune, neurological and endocrine systems of people dealing with CF/FM. There is also damage to the cells which causes the cells to become hormone resistant, insulin resistant and which interferes with the cells ability to produce energy within the mitochondria. I can't think of anything that might be more traumatic for people to deal with other than leprosy, cancer or an orphan disease. Ignorance and outright denial have caused a hugh amount of suffering to many people.

Leprosy caused people to be cast out of society and these poor souls were left to literally rot. We now know that it was a bacteria that caused this condition. I always felt there was a biological explanation for this condition and that when it was found those who were responsible for these people's fates would have a lot of karma to deal with if not in this life then in the next!

The sad thing about FM/CF is the many years of denial that there was such a thing as leaky gut syndrome. They claimed if someone truly had this they wouldn't be alive! A good excuse for harming so many with toxic, dangerous, overly prescribed drugs and exposing people to toxic substances? You be the judge! Of course I hope you read the whole book before you decide!

It was very frustrating that the doctors I saw could not tell me what caused my fibromyalgia or worse they couldn't tell me what to do for it. My treating physician said "there is no cure for fibromyalgia; you'll just have to learn to live with it." I of course knew that there was no living with the amount of pain and lack of ability to function that I was experiencing.

The fact that I had so much pain now in the neck and shoulder from being re-injured only compounded the problem. I was off work for a number of months and thought maybe I was feeling better and I would try to do light duty. I had to convince my physician to even let me try this. I should have listened to him and not even have tried it. I sat at a desk and did inspection. They wouldn't even allow me to lift a small bin weighing no more than 10 lbs. After sitting for just one hour, I knew I was in trouble, I had pain first in the neck and shoulder which progressed to the whole upper body, then to the whole body.

I wasn't able to sleep at all by the end of a week of this for by now the pain I had seemed to be everywhere. I knew of course that there was something very seriously wrong, but I didn't know yet how much was wrong. I was then taken back off from work by the orthopedic surgeon. He said he could see spam in my neck muscles when he did an X-ray at the hospital. He then took me back off from work and said I would not be returning to work.

After your disabled for a year, you are terminated from your employment. The insurance company said they would refer me to a lawyer that had helped others obtain their disability for fibromyalgia/chronic fatigue but they changed their mind after they were given the information that they video taped me picking up small pinecones. The social security judge I had at my first hearing used the fact that I tried to return to work to say I proved I could do this job. I think this was ridiculous since obviously they wouldn't let me lift anything. My physician wrote social security twice saying I was permanently and totally disabled. They ignored this. I was lead to believe he agreed I could return to work, when in fact he wrote two opinions in my soc. sec. file that I was permanently disabled. They also of course knew I had to take anodynos from the nurse to be able to even sit for 8 hours. This is the common harassment people on worker's comp experience. My physician said, "don't take it personally they do it to everyone." Of course it was personal; I was totally debilitated by this time. Of course, all of this is evident in my records which I encourage anyone in a similar situation to ask for from their insurance company. By law they are required to give it to you when you write and request this information. However, don't be surprised if they give you excuses and try to get out of giving it to you. I requested my employee records but they said they couldn't find them. When we had a hearing they had found them.

MY EXPERIENCES

I learned that there was a physician nearby that had fibromyalgia himself. I asked my treating physician to set up an appointment with him. Since this doctor had this condition himself; I thought he might know more than the doctors I had been seeing. I would learn later that worker's comp sends a lot of people with fibromyalgia to him. I however was on long term disability not worker's comp.

When I arrived in his office, he came in the room wearing shoes that had cushioned soles with at least a couple inches of extra rubber to pad his feet. I thought I hope I don't end up with that much pain in my feet that I have to wear shoes like that!

He gave me some literature on fibromyalgia. I feel it might be eye opening to share the contents of some of this information with you the readers. It sheds some light on how little was actually known and how much has been learned in the last 10 years. This information follows:

Occupational Issues:

I recently completed a research project on FM in the work place. Our research has shown that the best tolerated occupations appear to be those which involve an environmentally stable in-door, warm, non-drafty work location and a job which involve the performance of light variable activities (seated, some standing & walking with varied tasks during the work day). FM factory workers may have significant problems with assembly line work and seem to be more prone to superimposed environmental and emotional stresses. Workers with FM seem be more likely to develop repetitive motion syndromes because we are much less likely to relax our muscles even during rest periods than other workers or because our muscles and tendons are "just not as good" as non-fibromyalgic individuals. Like it or not, our muscles just aren't as good as "normal individuals". Recent reports from Europe and Oregon have shown that FM workers have less strength and endurance than "normal" individuals when placed in testing programs. Rotating shift work is especially hard our our problem with sleep disturbance. When possible I encourage FM patients to work a day shift. (typed as presented in information). My comment: (Keep in mind a lot of people with FM will progress to CF especially if they are under a lot of stress or they have had toxic exposures.)

Physical Stressors:

Factors that aggravate FM include working in one place with arms suspended above the work surface, repetitive activities, and remaining in one position for a prolonged period of time whether it's sitting, standing, or even driving. Acute infections are stressors that often produce profound aggravation of symptoms of FM. Fibromyalgia is also very closely related to a condition called Chronic Fatigue Syndrome: some physicians feel that the two conditions are somehow related, but there definite clinical features and chemical research studies that differentiate between the two. Both conditions feature fatigue as a major symptom but CFS patients also have good clinical evidence of a chronic or relapsing infectious process as the triggering event. Most individuals with FM experience similar reactions to specific activities: we just do not tolerate holding our muscles in a sustained isometric position for prolonged period of time whether it's typing, playing the piano. Doing assembly line work, operating a vacuum sweeper or cooking at home. Sustained contraction of the shoulder muscles to support our arms in front of us tends to produce pain in the neck, upper back and shoulders that gradually builds and spreads up and down the back. We can do heavy work as long as it is not repetitive. (Questionable) Working rotating shifts at work has been reported as an aggravating factor by many of my patients, perhaps because of the aggravation of their sleep disturbance. (We now know toxins from chemicals and metals cause leaky gut and definitely play a role according to leading research.)

The Cure of Fibromyalgia (Etiology):

Current research has shown there are most likely several biochemical or structural defects which predispose us to develop Fibromyalgia some time during our lives. The defects are probably there from birth, and like so many non-lethal biochemical defects, often becomes symptomatic in early adulthood. Recent studies have shown that there are chemical abnormalities in the central nervous system of individuals with fibromyalgia. Current research is centered on (1) abnormalities of the brain: hypothalamus-pituitary-adrenal axis. (2) Alteration of neurotransmitter receptors in the brain and spinal cord. (3) Possible defects in the chemical pathway leading to the manufacture of Serotonin and other nervous system chemicals. (4) A deficiency of growth hormone secretion in the brain. (5) Abnormalities of substance P, a neuro-peptide, which is seen to be elevated in the spinal fluid of FM patients and thought to play a major role in chronic pain problems. (6) Abnormalities of high energy phosphate (ATP) in red blood cells. ATP is a fundamental chemical involved in energy transfer in the body. Chemical abnormalities are probably also involved in depression, psychiatric disorders and migraine headaches although there are definite differences between these conditions and FM. (We now know the physical causes aren't genetic.) (We now know prolonged pain plays a role in changing the chemical pathways that conduct pain signals to the brain leading to chronic pain syndromes.)

Treatment:

The most effective treatments for FM has been the use of the tri-cyclics, exercise, over the counter pain medications, and avoidance of the stress factors described above. (One Doctor's Opinion)

(Nsaids can lead to auto-intoxication from colon according to Dr. Gloria Gilbere N.D., D.A. Hom., Ph.D. in the Doctor's Prescription for Healthy Living/Volume 5, Number 5) who said she almost died from taking these drugs.) She recommends use of enzymes for these issues.

I used Effexor XR for several months and got to a place where I could not go to sleep. I was sleeping one to two hours a night. I went off this and gradually over several months started to be able to sleep. I used melatonin in place of the Effexor XR. I believe now that the cause of this was that my methylation system wasn't working properly due to toxic exposures and the drug was no doubt building up in my system. Metals and drugs can damage the P-450 enzyme that helps the liver detox. My caffeine challenge also showed an imbalance in the liver detox pathways.

Unfortunately the specialist with FM giving me the advice to take ibuprofen and aspirin only worsened my condition. This only made my pain explode and I'm sure added to the leaky gut syndrome. I would never advise anyone to take NSAID's, they will only aggravate the problem. I only took them very conservatively at that. I now know there are enzymes, herbs and supplements that address the problems associated with this condition without the side affects of irritation to the intestinal tract. No wonder he was walking around on thickly padded shoes!

I meet a lady through the fibromyalgia support group that had been injured in the service. They told her to take a lot of aspirin. She took so much that it broke down her intestinal tract and stomach lining. When I met her she could not get out of bed. She was being treated by the veteran's administration. She shared with me that she had around 50 spots on the liver where the liver tissues had died. She was taking a lot of medication.

She had a lot of food intolerances and she was in terrible pain most of the time. I asked her if she might like to try the course I had been on which had helped me and she said she would. She eliminated gluten and dairy, two of the foods that seem to be the worst offenders for people with leaky gut syndrome. I asked her to try and eat more whole live foods like fruits and vegetables. She saw some improvement with this course of action. I shared my essential oils of lavender and lemon which also seem to help.

I then introduced her to a product called colostrum which a friend shared with me. She found this to be a great help with pain and sleep. After about a week her pain level came down and she said she was sleeping better. I don't think anyone can comprehend how much stress it can create in one's body when you are disabled and under financial, emotional and physical stress. This leaches over in to the spiritual aspects of a person's life as well. It can eat away at the spirit like a malignant tumor or cancer. It made my spiritual life much stronger as it gave me time to study my bible and this opened up a new world which now allows me to see with new eyes what is going on in the world and it isn't a pretty picture right now! I believe we are at a critical junction where human, civil and personal rights are being threatened by the laws and people who should be protecting society.

She continued to see improvement with this product. Colostrum is the pre-milk the cow produces after a calf is born. It contains many things that help with the healing process. It has IGF-l growth factor that speeds healing along with interferon which helps a sluggish immune system. This should not be taken indefinitely because of these two elements which might over stimulate the immune system if taken for a prolonged period of time. It also has some antibody properties that fight invaders like bacteria and viruses. When cows are born they have an intestinal tract that hasn't fully matured. They have large spaces between the cells that will allow pathogens to get into their system. If calves are deprived of the colostrum for too long; they will not survive their first few days of life, it is that vital to their survival.

My husband and I had the same experience as our friends; the colostrum brought us to a certain level after which it did not seem to help. I believe the reason for this is because he was dealing with mercury toxicity and I was dealing with many heavy metals I could have only gotten from work. We both were dealing with a sluggish methylation system. This involves the detoxification pathways of the liver.

They are now using a drug called Rutuximab with people with a diagnosis of CF, rheumatoid arthritis and some cancers. I have read it contains monoclonal antibodies. I read one report by a physician that said all veterans were exposed to mycoplasmas in the vaccines. I haven't been able to confirm this but it is very possible. They now test every batch of vaccines for mycoplamas. You can find more information on this from Dr. Stan Montieth on Radio Liberty.com. A high percentage of soldiers seem to develop walking pneumonia after being given vaccines. It has also been said by many functional medicine physicians that mercury leads to leaky gut. Could there be a connection? I believe there definitely is, just read what Dr. Zoltan P. Rona says about leaky gut on his website. He has been treating these conditions for many years and he knew about this long before most physicians here in the United States.

CASES I'VE BEEN FAMILIAR WITH

We introduced a friend to colostrum and it really turned her situation around. I read that one of the pharmaceutical companies was trying to find a way to produce a drug from the properties in the colostrum because they found it to have many beneficial properties. There is a product on the market my physician told me contains antibodies and I wonder if it came from colostrum. I asked if he thought this is where they got the antibodies and he said probably.

Of course drugs are made with herbs that have been chemically altered, but now that they are finding nutrients can resolve many health issues they want to label nutrients as drugs. If this in deed happens, I'm afraid that the products will become so expensive that the average person will not be able to afford them. I do however believe that they should meet standards for purity. Many of the pharmaceuticals are now producing supplements themselves.

Another friend I met at a support group meeting had been dealing with CF/FM after an automobile accident. She became totally disabled. She had to have two knee replacements. She had been a secretary for one of the local schools. She started on colostrums and MSM and was amazed that her viral load seemed to just disappear. She asked to be retested to be sure the test was correct. She thought she had picked up these viruses due to a blood transfusion after her accident. She said she took her products to the hospital when she had her knee replacements and the nurses wanted to know what she was taking so she shared the information with them. When she told them how much help they had given her, they told her to keep taking the products.

In one of Dr. Cheney's reports he stated, "eventually we'll have recombinant nerve growth factors available." "Some are in testing stages now." "But I think this is where we'll be going in stage 3 of the illness, is bringing back this injured brain." "Because if we don't do that, they may be over the miser stage but they'll be locked into pretty significant functional impairment." "There will be things they'll never be able to do again." I asked my holistic doctor who was doing chelation about recombinant nerve growth factor availability and she said she didn't think this would ever be approved for treatment here in Indiana.

My friend and I who have traveled this road together for years have discussed this so many times, we just wonder if people's brains are functioning normally. I read one comment by a physician that possibly the toxins in our environment are having an impact and causing some of the aberrant behaviors we are seeing today. It surely is something to consider. It might help explain why children are acting out in a much more violent way. I never heard of children gunning down classmates when I was growing up. I think the violence in the video games might also be programming minds to become numb to violence. It might also explain some of the laws that have recently been passed by our lawmakers.

As a child I was always very healthy. I never had any of the childhood diseases other than croup. I was exposed to chicken pox when my step sisters came down with them, but all I experienced was a few bumps on my fingers. I really noticed a downturn in my health when I did the lead soldering job with my former employer. I had unrelenting fatigue after this which lead up to my shoulder injury. I had many routine tests which didn't show a thing. Of course most standard blood tests don't show anything when your dealing with FM/CF or metal exposures. I also had tests for cancer which were negative. I knew something was wrong but no one did the correct tests.

They used a lot of chemicals in their manufacturing processes as well as having soldering, welding and assembly operations. After I had worked for them for a few years, we had a meeting and we were told that they had gotten rid of some of their most dangerous chemicals, I was taken back. I never really thought about the fact that some of the things I might have been exposed to could be so toxic.

I did have trouble with one operation where there was a cement glue which was used to secure a lid on the product. I experienced dizziness, heart palpitations and severe fatigue which would not go away. I did get a physician's note that said I could not work in the area where this glue was used. They did not want to accept this. I was told they would be accepting liability if they did accept it. I refused to do this job and said I would have to quit if that was all they had for me to do. When I found the hazard sheet which was well out of sight, it cautioned that this chemical could cause asphyxiation with excessive exposure. They then moved me off this job.

I would say that if anyone has this kind of reaction to a chemical they are working with; they could be having a reaction to it and should ask to be removed from the area or be given some kind of protective gear so they are not breathing it. It was ventilated, but obviously this was not sufficient to prevent me from reacting to it. We now know that some chemicals can damage the DNA which can lead to cancer. We need to be very vigilant to limit any exposure to chemicals as well as heavy metals. With the ever increasing number of toxic chemicals in our environment this is a daunting task for all of us today. Maybe we should ask why there needs to be so many new and varied chemicals. I believe it is time that we put the welfare of the many before the profits of the few.

EUROPEAN STANDARDS

In Europe they have to prove a chemical is safe before they are allowed to add it to a product for human use. We seem to be far behind Europe in protecting the welfare of consumers. I believe instead of a profit driven society the demand will be going forward to be a consumer friendly profit driven society. I believe consumers are much more savvy thanks to people like Oprah and Dr. Oz.

We are reading that babies being born today already have over 200 known chemicals in their little bodies. It has also been stated that many people are born with lead already in their bones. I don't think they know how many heavy metals they may have but exposing them to any toxic metal such as mercury is beyond my understanding or comprehension.

There is a movement going on to ask the CDC what they have known about mercury in vaccines. Will we get the answers or will this just be another issue that goes away? Or worse, will congress allow them to pass a law that does away with the Freedom of Information Act.

I just read that there is a group called the "UN Environmental Programme."

Here is some information quoted from their website:

"In February 2009, the Governing Council of UNEP agreed on the need to develop a global legally binding instrument on mercury."

"The work to prepare this instrument is undertaken by an intergovernmental negotiating committee supported by the Chemicals Branch of the UNEP Division of Technology, Industry and Economics as secretariat." "The goal is to complete the negotiations before the twenty-seventh regular session of the Governing Council/Global Ministerial Enviornment Forum in 2013."

Recently President Obama and Eric Holder expressed sentiment that we should have an open government but there is a move to pass a law that would do away with the Freedom of Information Law which requires them to produce any document you might request. It's obvious they say one thing but do another! They could of course say they don't keep records back that far or that they just can't find any records. This is what I experienced when I ask OSHA for any records they might have on fumes produced on lead soldering that might have been done where I worked. The company claimed they had a test from 1990 the time frame in which I was still an employee. I think we need laws requiring OSHA to keep records for no less than 30 years on any toxic substances. Lead of course can remain in the bone for 30 years.

I would however find a material safety data sheet from the manufacturer that said specifically that solder melts at 100 degrees farenheight and gives off toxic lead and antimony at that level. The company I worked for claimed that there were no fumes given off because they melted the solder at such a low level. I think we have to believe the manufacturer, especially since the employer said in a letter earlier that there were very low fumes, not that there were no fumes. Research on OSHA's site would also indicate there are fumes from lead soldering operations.

Obviously there are fumes but the really significant thing I learned is that lead, antimony and other elements can be absorbed through the skin, this is specifically stated by the manufacturer of the soldering material. We weren't given gloves or the material safety data sheet. The material safety data sheet I later found after my denial of compesation states very specifically that elements in lead solder can be absorbed through the skin!

I also have a letter to senator Jim Hughes which I gave my lawyer signed by 4 co-workers who had also done this job. This senator by the way never responoded to this letter. This specifically states that we weren't given any gloves or the material safety data sheet while on this job. Obviously we were exposed due to the company's inattention to the hazard information. This was either not submitted as requested or ignored by the industrial commission.

OSHA STANDARDS

When the company claimed I said I got this from fumes, I said, "even if there were no fumes I believe you could be exposed through skin exposure." I also said, "I know lead can be absorbed and obviously the other elements can as well." I didn't have the material safety data sheet that says explicitly this can be absorbed through the skin at the time of hearing. I did have the Material Safety Data Sheet from the manufacturer that said gloves were required and the employer was required to monitor the breakthrough time on those gloves. This should have been in the record as well as my statements. This is why I believe all court hearings should have a court monitor which is required to record all statements made by a claimant. This was obviously not done! My lawyers were remiss in allowing this to go to the civil court judge without this information. The civil court judge was remiss in ignoring the Supreme Court Toxic Tort laws on the discovery rule! This states your time to sue does not start until you learn something the employer did exposed you to a toxic substance. The Supreme court said what they did might be considered malpractice but they didn't think it unethical!

Under Hazard Data they state:

"Route of entry: skin"
"Route of Entry: Inhalation"
"Route of Entry: Ingestion"
"Health Hazards—Acute and Chronic".

Obviously this proves where my exposures to these metals came from. This was however denied by worker's comp. They stated that since there were no fumes from the soldering operation, I couldn't have been exposed through this operation. They stated "there is no evidence that Elaine had exposure to lead while working at her employer and certainly did not have lead levels that are any different from persons in the general population." "She does not have an excess body burden of lead and does not have any evidence of lead toxicity." The Doctor's Data laboratory who did the previous IV chelation challenge determined that I had three times the elevated limits per the reference population for lead. OSHA research indicates my levels to be considered serious. Metals can insight the immune system for years. There is no way to measure the amount that is in the bones. You have to have more treatments than I was able to have to get it out and it is questionable if you ever get it out. Remember lead remains in the bone for 30 or more years. Lead is dangerous because it can re-immerge in the blood under times of stress or trauma. It also can affect the function of the thyroid, adrenals and other organs such as the liver and kidneys. New rules are asking that the amount of exposure limits be lowered. The rules related to allowable limits per the world health organization do not exceed 10 pg/dl.

Tests For Lead

There is a lawsuit going on against, Doctor's Data v. (quackwatch guy) Steven Barrett who claims the laboratory that does the urine analysis for physicians doing chelation is doing tests that aren't accurate. "Scientific Review of Alternative an Aborrant Medicine" was sued in California and the courts there ruled that no court of law should use his information in any hearing state or federal agency because they found him to not be credible. It will be interesting to see how this turns out. His information was used by my employer in my hearing. They suggested anyone doing chelation therapy is on the fringe of medicine. Let us remember that this therapy has been approved by the FDA for lead poisoning since World War II when sailors became toxic from painting the hulls of ships.

He of course not only has discredited Doctor's Data but the doctors doing chelation therapy. I believe this is part of an ongoing attack against practitioners who practice this kind of medicine. I would probably have been dead a long time ago had I not had some chelation. There is no way to know all the long term affects of this exposure. I have heard other people who were told they needed open heart surgery say they felt so much better after having chelation therapy and that they didn't feel they would have had the first surgery had they known about it. I have read that they are doing clinical trials to see if chelation is affective in heart disease. I wonder if we will get these results or if this will become obscure information from the public like so many other studies.

I had a hair analysis but have learned that some metals may not be present until the cells become healthy enough to release them. Also when one element is high others may not be showing. I have also learned that lead can go up and down as you chelate it and if there are other toxic elements that are high it might not show up on one test but be high on the next test. You may not be able to see all the toxic exposures on a hair analysis because the hair only shows what has been recently released by the cells. Cells will only release toxins when they become healthy enough to do so. If you have been nutrient deficient for a while this might interfere with a test result. It took 8 months of nutritional therapy for bismuth to be released when it was released it was off the chart, but other things weren't showing to be high. I would later find antimony showing in a nutritional evaluation blood test that didn't show in the hair analysis.

For lead poisoning to develop, prior acute exposures to lead need not occur. The body accumulates the metal over a lifetime, so even small doses added over a period of time (like being exposed over 8 mo. on the job) can cause lead poisoning. This is what I found when I did the research. I also found an article by The Agency For Toxic Disease Registry that stated that a person that has elevated levels for antimony got it from work. There is very little amounts of antimony in soil so it would be hard to pick it up from the environment. Antimony is one of the elements in lead soldering. The physician who found it in 2004 asked where I could have gotten this. I also had high levels of copper and beryllium, tin and bismuth all elements of the soldering material. I didn't have a clue I had all this at the time since I didn't know all the elements I had been exposed to. The first chelation specialist failed to give me all the test results. He did however tell me I had high levels of mercury and arsenic. You should always ask for all test results. I have since learned that arsenic is used to bind metals together in lead solders. I also have been in correspondence with a senator here in Indiana and he tells me that people working for pressure control devices and therm-o-stat switches are routinely exposed to mercury. No doubt this is because they handle the rolled steel arms which go into the product. I did a lot of this myself, this would account for some of the mercury exposure, cadmium, lead and arsenic.

The physician that found the antimony said, "It gets deep into the muscle tissue and causes the muscle to be weak." I can believe this since standing for 4 hours when I attempted to work put me in bed for two days with severe muscle spasm up and down my back.

He also stated that chelation might not get it out but it was worth a try to get some of it out. Antimony is a known carcinogen. I didn't know at this point all the metal exposures I was dealing with because the previous doctor failed to give me all the test results. Again you should always ask for any and all test results from your physicians. Some of this antimony would even show up in a nutritional evaluation test many years later. Of course I haven't had any help with all these very expensive tests, nutritional therapy and treatment because they denied my case.

I am still dealing with effects of the metals. After the last chelation I developed pyrroles in the blood and my methylation was off so I had a bad reaction to the chelation. I was experiencing a lot of auto-immune symptoms. I had a lump come up on top of my left foot and it was so painful it felt like the tendon above the big toe might burst. I also had a lump come up on my left wrist. My wrist was so painful I couldn't use it for a few days. I am now trying to correct the methylation problem. I believe any physician doing chelation should first check the patient's nutritional status and the status of the methylation system before attempting to do chelation on the patient. I was put on an advanced methylating product which only caused the condition to become worse. I developed a lot of pain everywhere. I found a product by Dr. Cartwright which has reduced glutathione and cysteine in it. I started taking this and my pain came down 50% in the first week. I am now taking Cellgevity from Max International and this product has a proprietary patented formula which helps the cells produce their own glutathione. This has been a Godsend as I am experiencing less inflammation and an increase of a sense of wellbeing. By raising the glutathione, you help the cells produce ATP within them. This is why people get an increase in their energy when they start on this product. My husband went from needing a nap after working out at the YMCA to not needing a nap and having energy until 10 or 11 PM.

There is good information that I found on low glutathione being related to the methylation block associated with chronic fatigue syndrome. This information can be found on the internet when you do a search. The researchers name is Richard von Konynenburg. He also has a video on U-Tube regarding this information.

Like I stated earlier, lead stays in the bones and tissue for 30 or more years. It can be released when a person is under severe stress or develops metabolic changes such as leaky gut syndrome. I found a research article that stated when lead gets stirred up in the blood it can lead to M.S. That means we are all at risk for developing a neurological disease. This also means as our environment becomes more polluted from burning of coal these elements being released will be more of a health hazard. It is a shame that the laws put in place to put scrubbers on the chemineys of coal burning and manufacturing facilities were not implemented years ago. I talked with a lady who lived within a mile of a plant and she was very ill with CF/FM. According to what I have read, nickel and uranium exposure can continually activate the immune system indefinitely. I believe this may also be true for mercury since it and other metals deplete the glutathione from the body. Glutathione helps rid the body of toxins and free radicals.

RESEARCH SOURCES

A good research article was found on Pub Med. This is a publication of research from around the world and I recommend that anyone looking for good research use this site which is government sponsored. Their study on "Skin absorption of inorganic lead (PbO) and the effect of skin cleansers" states that PbO powder can pass through the skin and that skin decontamination done after 30 minutes of exposure did not decrease skin absorption occurring over 24 hours and stresses the need to prevent skin contamination when using toxic substances."

Another article found on Pub Med under "Precutaneous absorption of inorganic lead compounds" states "the amount of lead on the dorsal hand was significantly correlated with the amount in the blood" after testing was done. This was a lead battery manufacturer.

In an article called "Parental occupational lead exposure and lead concentration of newborn cord blood" they state, "there were significant differences between the non-exposed and the maternal exposure groups, and also between the non-exposed and paternal groups." "All 26 maternal exposures were from lead soldering operations." In other words they found elements in the cord blood from the lead soldering of pregnant mothers. "I think this leaves no doubt this operation exposes you to the elements in the soldering material, especially if gloves are not given."

The Bell companies once did a lot of lead soldering and I found research they had done in an article which stated "vapors generated at any pressure can be inhaled of course, contributing to potential health problems."

People who used solder to seal plumbing pipes have had this exposure referred to as plumerism. The only reason I can think of for this is that it was common knowledge that they had been exposed to lead.

Symptoms of Lead Exposure

Interestingly the symptoms of lead exposure are pain in the muscles and connective tissues, headaches etc. These are the same symptoms of fibromyalgia.

Here is a list from the CDC if you have lead levels at levels between 20-39pg/dl:

Spontaneous abortion
Reduced newborn birth weight
Possible blood pressure changes
Possible renal dysfunction
Possible non-specific Symptoms:

HEADACHE, FATIGUE, SLEEP DISTURBANCES, CONSTIPATION, DIARRHEA, ARTHRALGIA, MYAGLIA, DECREASED LIBIDO, MOOD SWINGS, PERSONALITY CHANGES, CNS (central nervous system) EFFECTS, MEMORY AND ATTENTION DEFICITS

10-29 pg/dl This (mid-teens) has been the estimated exposure from lead gasoline in the general public in the 70's and early 80's.) Maybe it is all the pollution that is causing so many more pre-mature births than usual.

Possible spontaneous abortion
Reduced newborn birth weight
Possible blood pressure changes
Possible renal dysfunction

In the 70's and early 80's people had blood lead levels in the mid teens according to an article I recently read. This was also stated by Dr. Gary Gordon on a recent video he made for the internet. Dr. Gordon is the physician who did testing for heavy metals before he sold his business to Doctor's Data who now does testing for physicians who do chelation. I am sure he has seen these tests. When lead was removed from gasoline the lead levels dropped to 1 or 2 pg/dl. But remember lead remains in the bones for 30 years and with additional exposure it can tip you in to lead poisoning.

Lead can also re-immerge in the blood under times of stress and trauma. Maybe a lot of lead poisoning is being mislabeled as fibromyalgia. Dr. Cheney stated that these people are full of chemicals and toxins and have to be detoxed to see results. Of course we women are exposed to more chemicals in our personal care products, make-up, cologne etc. Some people claim to rid themselves of fibromyalgia by taking more magnesium. If this is the case, I believe they had a nutrient deficiency not full blown fibormyalgia or chronic fatigue. I have read that magnesium does give some protective qualities to tissues exposed to metals. Dr. Gordon stated that many people with high lead levels have committed suicide. I can believe that this is true!

Toxins such as mercury and lead are particularly dangerous and can suppress the thyroid function. They also impair the detoxification process and lead to water and fat accumulation. In the beginning of my illness I kept on putting on weight and didn't know why since I hadn't changed my eating habits. In the mornings my hands and face would seem particularly puffy.

CHEMICAL SENSITIVITIES AND CHEMICAL EXPOSURES

I remember having a reaction to a co-workers smoke while I was still working. At one time they allowed smoking on the job. Since this person sat across from me her smoke would come my way. I remember getting up one morning and my eyes were almost swollen shut. To this day I can't tolerate being in a smoking environment. I believe when you are toxic from chemicals or metals it makes you more reactive to your environment. Having been exposed to bio-toxins may also mimic other toxic exposures. Bio-toxins can be anything from mold to bacteria or parasite.

I also can't stand going down the laundry detergent isle of the grocery store or smelling heavy perfume on anyone. Even smelling fabric softener in clothes recently laundered will cause some nose and throat irritation. By the way, I have read that some laundry softeners have chemicals which could be harmful to the body. Shame on the companies that produce products which they know contain toxic chemicals! I have read stories of mothers who observed their families allergies going away after eliminating fabric softeners from their laundry. I know these products would cause my skin to itch. My husband and I are even sensitive to what laundry detergent we use and have had the best luck with Meleluca and Shaklee products.

You can make your own fabric softener. Just add 8 Cups white vinegar and 1 and l/4 cup warm water in a bucket, add 1 cup baking soda and stir constantly (mixture will fizz).

Pour this into a clean gallon size jug add 1 tsp. essential oil (lavender or thieves) add 1/2 cup to rinse cycle. This will help you avoid chemicals in softener products and save your family money.

Lead in the blood can lead to pyrroles which cause pain in hands, feet and muscles. Lead can also lead to anemia of the blood because it interferes with the synthesis of heme the human hemoglobin necessary for oxygen transport. Lead also interferes with normal cellular calcium metabolism. Because calcium and calcium-binding proteins serve as the messengers for many basic cellular processes, even small amounts of lead can do damage.

Welding processes also produce many toxins. This might include toxic gases like ozone or nitrogen oxides, or intense hazards such as untraviolet radiation. Processes involving stainless steel, cadmium, or lead-coated steel, and metals such as nickel, chrome, zinc, and copper are of particular concern. These fumes may be more toxic than fumes encountered when welding iron or mild steel.

Unfortunately I know of people I worked with that also developed severe health issues. One of my dear friends became ill about the same time I did. She started with carpel tunnel in both wrists. This pain progressed to her neck and then body pain. She had all the same symptoms as I did so I have kept in touch with her all these years. She was diagnosed with dysotonomia. Dysotonomia is just another name for fibromyalgia. I have shared much of my research with her. She was sent to physicians who gave her a lot of pain medications. Some of these can cause auto-intoxication of the colon. They blamed her carpel tunnel on her thyroid condition so they refused to give her compensation for it. I learned that she had been exposed to a soft lead soldering material. She worked dropping small parts into this substance all day for many months. She was out ill for a couple of days and said when she came back to work they were told they had to use gloves. They were given thin surgical gloves that she said got holes after about a half hour of use. Obviously this did not serve the purpose of skin protection.

Unfortunately for her, her husband would also become disabled. He had worked for a manufacturer of bus seats. He worked in an area where the foam for the seats was glued. My sister worked there also. She said when you walked by that area the fumes would almost bowl you over. He has a cyst on his kidney but the V.A. can't tell him what it is. They are living on fixed incomes with help from a son who lives with them. She can not afford to have testing or chelation treatments. I have watched as her condition continues to deteriorate. She has high blood pressure and many health challenges. She suffers from daily pain and fatigue. My heart just aches for her since I know that not addressing these issues properly will only lead to worsening of her conditions. She takes vitamin C and tries to eat right as well as possible on a fixed income. She says when she drinks more juices and eats certain foods she experiences more symptoms. In a righteous world she would have had disability early on and been able to get the help she needed which should include chelation and supplementation.

One unfortunate young lady worked over a chemical bath where she checked parts. She developed a tumor behind her eye. She had the eye removed and a glass eye replacement. When she came back to work she was placed back on this operation. She had problems with the eye watering and the tumor came back. Unfortunately she died from her cancer.

I recently learned that one employee who worked in an area they called the pouring room is now in an assisted living facility. She has Alzheimer. There were many fumes in this area. I worked in there for two days. I told the supervisor if I had problems I would let her know since they had the same chemical I had reacted to earlier. She had asked if I thought I could work in there. I had a toxic headache for two days from smelling these chemicals. When I told the supervisor I had a toxic headache for two days, she took me out of this area. This area was not ventilated at one time. I spoke with an employee who went back to school for nursing. She said she made a report to OSHA about this and the problem was corrected. She said she was having some health problems she thought might be related to exposures on this job.

Of course those who do chelation will tell you metals can lead to heart disease, circulatory problems and a long list of health issues. I found one report that said metals cause auto-immune conditions in the body. I believe chemicals also act in the same way. Antibodies chasing antigens in the system can do damage to the blood vessel linings causing fibrin and plaque to form to address this damage. This plague can become unstable, break off and cause a stroke or heart attack. Functional medical doctors use vitamin K2 to help break down this plague and reverse heart disease. Also nattokinase will break down fibrin and help prevent heart attack and stoke. Nattokinase is a soy based enzyme. Like many products on the market, some may be more effective than others.

I met a young man in chelation therapy who worked as a steel worker. He said his job was to roll the sheets of metal that we used in our therm-o-stat manufacturing. He said he was full of cancer from lead, arsenic, mercury, cadmium etc. He said he enjoyed his job and would do it again. He also shared with me that he had to fight worker's comp for a long time before they agreed to pay for his treatments. I have had no help because they denied my claim saying I signed off in 1996 when I settled the shoulder injury. This I believe is an example of a miscarriage of justice since it ignores the toxic tort rules in that state. I wrote the Department of Labor and they advised me to write my senators and governor of Ohio. I have written several letters and had no response. I was told to contact the attorney general, again no response. Recently I viewed a video of Senator Kucinich saying that workers have lost their rights and people were also losing their human rights in Ohio and this needed to be changed. I wrote him and it was marked out for delivery but has not been documented delivered as of this writing. When I wrote senator Sawyer it was returned months later marked undeliverable. I don't know why any piece of mail should take months to be returned to sender. I have read that senators in Ohio have been unresponsive to their constituents. I don't understand this but there does seem to be something going on that doesn't seem quite right.

I have spent a fortune of my own money trying to get well. People who have long retention of metals have a harder time getting well. Many metals will cause a senergistic effect which will also complicate your recovery, especially if the liver has been affected and the methylation system is down. These problems need to be addressed before you attempt to do chelation, otherwise you may get a bad result. This was my experience with my last chelation treatment. I experienced an immune system that evidently over-reacted because the metylation was not working properly. I was also dealing with some nutritional deficiencies no doubt caused by the binding of enzymes by these metals. Lead can also have a direct affect on the intestinal tract. I developed pyrroles in the blood which can cause pain in the hands, feet and muscles. It also causes severe anxiety and depression. I also have had a severe B-12 deficiency which lead to symptoms that mimicked a heart attack. I had pain that went through the chest into the back around the ribs, up in to the throat and jaw. My physician says everyone dealing with fibromyalgia has a problem in the first pathway of the methylation system. This is probably due to the fact that metals bind up enzymes that carry nutrition to the cells. Mercury can lead to a B-12 deficiency.

Approximately 20% of the concentration of lead that can cause death can cause cognitive disturbances such as reduced attention span and memory, learning disabilities and lowered IQ's. It also lowers growth hormone in children. In developing countries it has been estimated that 80% of children 3-5 are believed to have blood levels exceeding health standards set by WHO (World Health Organization). I have also read WHO controls what vaccines will be given. China is adding many coal burning facilities and I'm reading their cities are very polluted. One physician recently stated that much of our mercury is coming from their coal burning. We have enough of our own pollution, we shouldn't have to deal with everyone else's pollution.

In July 2006 the EU ruled that heavy metals be banned from all kinds of electrical and electronic goods including refrigerators computers and vacuum cleaners. I wondered what they had replaced lead-tin solder with. I spoke with someone who worked for another company doing the old soldering; they weren't given gloves. She said the company replaced this with something new they said was better for the employees. She shared with me that when she had a colonoscopy and they administered sedatives her heart stopped and they had to restart it. I wonder if all those years of exposure weakened her heart or made her more reactive to the drugs. I do believe metals make you more reactive to chemicals and drugs. Lead can act directly on the gut. I share these stories to impress upon the readers how dangerous being exposed to lead and other toxins can be and how much damage it can cause to the body. I also share this because we have and are still being exposed to metals in our environment.

ENDOGENOUS TOXINS

Endogenous toxins are toxins of metabolism of which the body must rid itself. There is some recent research that indicates metals may interfere with this process when the methylation system becomes affected. Mercury for instance can bind up glutathione and deplete it from the detox processes of the body. This would allow toxins to build up in the system. It would also weaken the immune system as this process advances.

Exogenous toxins which come mainly from manufacturing, stop functioning of the enzymes which carry the nutrients to the cells, this is their toxic effect. This would explain why I was deficient in many trace minerals when I was given a hair analysis around 1995. I have heard comedians making jokes about metal exposures. They may not think it is so entertaining when they learn they themselves have been exposed to many toxins in their environment or if they themselves become affected by toxins.

TOXIC EFFECTS FROM METALS

Metals can affect the P450 enzyme in the liver which helps the liver detox. I had a caffeine liver challenge which indicated that I had an elevated caffeine clearance which is indicative of induced Phase I (cytochrome P450) activity. This can result in excess production of free radicals as well as biotranformed intermediate compounds which can exert their own toxic effects. This overactive state generally occurs as a result of exposure to endogenous or exogenous toxins. My glutathione peroxidase, however, was found depressed. This is an important front line enzyme of the antioxidant defense team. Lower levels of glutathione are associated with higher risk of oxidative damage in the body, and have been observed in disorders associated with free radicals, including alcoholism, cancer, atherosclerosis, rheumatoid arthritis and cataracts, and autism. Cancer rates are much higher in areas where selenium is not available in the soil. Also iodine is very scarce in the northeast part of the U.S.

My Phase I/PhaseII ratio for glucuronidation was elevated. A high ratio between Phase I and any of the Phase II pathways implies imbalanced detoxification in the body. The activated compounds, coming out of Phase I are potentially toxic and may accumulate, leading to illness. Eliminating excess toxin exposure, and supplying antioxidants as well as nutritional support for the Phase II pathways are critical to rebalancing of the system. A good form of absorbable folic acid along with B-12, B-6 and zink are essential.

Metals will cause an acidic condition in the body. You can check this by using the urine PH strips you find in the pharmacy. If you are dealing with metals you might consider taking 1,000 mg. vitamin C a day or 2,000-4000 vitamin D's. Of course if you are on a detox protocol you'll want to follow your doctor's recommendations.

There are many other conditions related to an acidic environment of the body a list follows:

Chronic fatigue syndrome
Weight gain
Joint pain
Aching muscles
Constipation
Urinary-tract problems
Stomach aches
Nausea kidney stones
And loss of vitality

Gastritis
Immune deficiency
Ulcers
Obesity
Diabetes
Osteopenia
Osteoporosis
Gout
Circulatory weakness

DIET AND AUTO-IMMUNE CONDITIONS

I believe grains should actually be a very small portion of our diet and for anyone with a gluten intolerance should be avoided like the plague. It has been said there are 300 different auto-immune symptoms associated with gluten intolerance. I believe that! I had pain from head to toe before I learned I head leaky gut and gluten and casein intolerance! I believe this was brought on by the drugs for the shoulder injury, trauma and metal exposures. I've had several celiac tests since which were negative. My titers to gliadin from gluten were off the charts when I was first tested. The doctor asked me how I walked into his office, I said, "very carefully." It is a shame no one had tested me for this earlier. After being on the colostrums, I was retested and my titers were under 10 however my symptoms did not go away. I was still dealing with pain and fatigue. This is when I started looking for other causes for my condition.

To alkalinize your diet you need to eat less read meat, decrease amount of fat you consume, eat few pasteurized dairy products, avoid white sugar, eat more fruits and vegetables. Eat more nuts, seeds and whole grains (unless sensitive). Use fresh lemon (l/2 lemon, pinch of stevia in 8oz water) is a great alkalinizer. I have used this frequently along with anti-oxidants and it really helps protect the cells from free radicals.

I just saw a video by Dr. Leonard Coldwell and he says anyone can get rid of cancer in a few days by alkalinizing the body. He recommends natural vitamin E, vitamin C 100 mgs. a day, l/2 tsp of sea salt in a gallon of water per day (unless counter-indicated). You need to alkalinize the body to 7.5 ph. A good way to do this is by using the Master Lemon Cleanse (l/2 lemon, pinch of Cheyenne and 1-2 tablespoons of pure Maple Syrup).

Intense physical exercise may lead to suppressed immune function that activates the stress response. This might explain why extreme athletes fall over from heart attacks when we think they should be in great shape.

Exercise activates serotonin and norepinephrine which lifts the mood. Walking seems to be the best exercise for anyone dealing with CF/FM. This is a gentle passive exercise that doesn't place too much stress on the joints.

OVERLOOKED TESTS FOR CF/FM

There are a number of tests which are sometimes overlooked but may be very important when dealing with CF/FM. You might ask for a C-reactive protein test which if high indicates an inflammatory response is going on. C-reactive protein is made in the liver in response to antigens (anything foreign) in the system.

If your homocysteine is too high this can indicate you are at risk for a heart attack.

For optimal blood pressure you need balanced levels of a gaseous molecule called Nitric Oxide. This is produced form argenine and oxygen. Nitric Oxide signals the blood vessels to relax. Dr. Oz recently recommended taking argenine for high blood pressure.

Chronic fatigue has been linked to viral infections such as the Epstein Bar, or environmental toxins. The CDC states that chronic fatigue is an end stage of a disease process. We now know that toxins and free radicals can damage the cells and the mitochondria within the cells that produce energy. The Montague/Hooper Paper of 2001 found that an enzyme that takes out viruses was damaged. They believe this was related to toxins in the system.

In the early 1990's doctors were being told that chronic fatigue/fibromyalgia were somato (all in your head) forms of illness. It is untold the amount of suffering this has caused. I know their have been many lives destroyed or lost due to this course of action.

Physical or emotional stress, which is commonly reported as a pre-onset condition in chronic fatigue syndrome patients, activates the lypothalamic-pituitary-adrenal axis leading to an increased release of cortisol and other hormones. Cortisol and corticotrophin releasing hormones influence the immune system and many other body systems. Dr. Cheney stated that there may be permanent damage within these systems if this condition is left untreated for too long.

Anxiety and worry only worsen the disease process by dampening the immune response and even raising cytokine production.

Fibromyalgia patients have exaggerated mast cell reactivity. This can be associated with irritable bowel syndrome, food sensitivities, inhalant allergies and interstitial cystitis. This explains some of the co-morbidity of FMS patients. Some of this may be reversed by healing the leaky gut and getting rid of the body's toxic load. Dr. Gordon stated on a recent video that everyone has leaky gut to some degree today!

Chronic stress response depletes important electron scavengers such as glutathione the important protector of mitochondrial and cellular mechanisms. Glutathione can also be depleted by low-dose chronic mercury intoxication along with other toxins.

Researchers have found pro-inflammatory cytokines elevated as much as four fold. Substance P (a pain conduction chemical), nerve growth factor and tumor necrosis factor-alpha appear to be active in the patho-physiology of the illness. Elevated cytokines may be caused by hormone imbalances, sleep deprivation and toxic exposures to chemicals and heavy metals. There is evidence for nutritional deficiencies; of course metals bind the enzymes that carry nutrients to the cells.

All of the neuro-transmitters are probably low. DHEA and natural progesterone in some cases have positive effect on dopamine levels. Many with chronic fatigue syndrome also have inhalant allergies.

Growth hormone may be deficient because of the sleep disturbances common in fibromyalgia. We produce growth hormone when we get into the deep rim sleep necessary for repair of body tissues. I am sure my inability to sleep after being injured and re-injured contributed to the development of the FM. I was lucky to sleep 1-2 hours a night, this went on for about 5 months. I have read that people who have gone without sleep for 5 months have died from their inability to sleep. This just shows how important getting a good nights sleep really is. I believe the IgF-1 growth hormone is produced during rem sleep.

SYMPTOMS OF CF/FM

You may experience feelings of numbness or tingling in parts of your body or poor circulation in some areas. Many people are very sensitive to odors, bright lights loud noises and medicines. You may also experience dry eyes and trouble focusing on nearby objects. Problems with dizziness and balance also may occur. Some have chest pain. A rapid or irregular heartbeat or shortness of breath. Headaches and jaw pain also are common.

Digestive symptoms include difficulty swallowing, heartburn, gas, cramping abdominal pain, and alternating diarrhea and constipation.

You may experience frequent urination and pain in the bladder. I believe this is caused because of the up-regulation of the immune system and increased cytokine production which causes inflammation. Some may have painful menstrual periods and painful sexual intercourse. Memory loss and mood disorders or depression and anxiety are the most frustrating of the symptoms.

I felt like I had been dumped into a dark tunnel which had no light and no way out! I learned in a bible study class that my name means "light" in Hebrew. When I had a visit with one of the nurse practitioners at my physician's office I shared some of my story with him. I said, "if my life does not amount to anything else, I hope I have been a little light to the world." His response was, "you have been more light than you even know."

I have shared much of the research in this book with this doctor's office. They said they never saw so much research in one place, but they were very appreciative of it and said they were glad for any and all information I could give them. How refreshing to find a true Christian doctor who is really interested in the welfare of his patients. I know he tries to keep up on all the latest information out there so he can really help his patients get well and stay well. He always spends the time he needs to find out what is going on from one visit to the next. If you don't have a physician like this

I suggest you go to a support group meeting and talk to people there to find out if there is anyone in your area like this. I said, you can see how desperate I was to find out what I was dealing with by all the research I have done.

I knew there were many others with the same misery. The only thing that kept me going was my determination to find some answers so I could get well and help others dealing with this. I decided to go to support group meeting to see if there might be a common tread among all the people with this condition. What I found was that most people had experienced a trauma, surgery or severe emotional upset. Having been prescribed many drugs was also a common thread. (See my information under leaky gut syndrome.)

Without proper treatment FMS can cause major disability as patients become unable to carry out normal activities. The longer a person is in pain, the more muscle damage is going on. FM undermines everything you are and can do. I felt like everything I once was had been sucked down into such profound darkness I couldn't find my way out. At my worst I could not get out of bed for a couple of weeks. I felt like each breath might be my last. The saddest thing I felt was that I might pass and no one would know what happened to me or why. I had so much inflammation that I could hardly move.

MY EXPERIENCES WITH CF/FM

It was like the life force was slowly being sucked out of my body. This came after dealing with social security and a very arrogant condescending judge. I was told that he was rough before I even went in there. He was most interested in asking me if I drank and how much I drank. He didn't ask about my symptoms or the condition. He looked at my lawyer and said this is "bull shit." I thought my heart was going to stop right then and there. My lawyer warned me to not say anymore than I had to because anything I said would be used against me. The lawyer answered "I know." Then later he claimed he did everything he could to defend my case! No wonder people don't trust lawyers! My spirit wasn't totally broken. This made me more determined to find the answers to this mysterious and disabling condition. I did file a complaint with the department of social security and I received an apology. They said they couldn't discipline judge because he had stepped down. I think that they probably had many complaints about him because my friend in Mass. asked me why they had so many people being denied their disability in my area.

The other humiliating thing I experienced was to be sent to a psychologist. He asked ridiculous questions that were on a personal level. I couldn't believe this. I don't think someone's sex life is anyone elses business! This should be a personal matter. I quess the only way this sort of thing changes is with enlightenment of people in higher places. The problem seems to be that most people are too intimidated to speak out about their experiences. I'm so tired of being told "you have to be careful what you say." "We don't have free speech anymore." This was from a para legal from second lawyers office! Where did our free speech go? Does anyone remember what Patrick Henry said? He said, "give me liberty or give me death." When this condition is in a flair up or is in the critic stages you feel like you have been handed a walking death sentence. How dare anyone treat another human being with such arrogant condescending actions. I think most people can only begin to imagine the mental strength it takes to deal with all of this, not only the condition but the condescending manner with which people have been treated.

OTHER PEOPLE EXPERIENCES

My friend in Arizona did not have experiences like this. She had Dr. Scott Rigden for a treating physician who wrote her a very comprehensive report and she had her disability in about 2 mo. Dr. Rigden was recognized as researcher of the year a couple years ago for CF/FM. Unfortunately there were no doctors in the area I lived that had a clue what I was dealing with and no one would help me. I did eventually find a Christian doctor who wrote me a great letter that helped me win my case. I had all the same symptomology my friend in Az. had.

I don't know what I would have done without an understanding spouse. He has had his own challenges with fatigue. We believe this came from the mercury released from his amalgams along with environmental exposures, no doubt. He has had trouble getting rid of this toxicity and chronic fatigue himself for many years. I think we now know why he has had these issues. Mercury is one of the leading causes of leaky gut syndrome. I believe his methylation system was also affected.

I prayed that the Lord would help me find some answers for all this misery. I went to my computer and prayed "Lord if you help me find the answers I promise I will help as many people as I can." I did about two clicks and I was in Dr. Zoltan P. Rona's website. He was talking about leaky gut syndrome and its connection to chronic fatigue syndrome/ fibromyalgia. Everything he said made so much sense. I knew I had found a key to unlocking this mysterious problem.

I have had some interesting experiences while traveling this rough and bumpy road called chronic fatigue/ fibromyalgia.

One of my friends developed these conditions after having a back injury while doing a double parallel bar loop. She missed the bar and fell backward on the matt. This resulted in actually breaking her back. She had three fractured vertebrae. She was in the middle of competition and like the trooper she is, she wanted to see her group compete more than she thought about taking care of herself. She had also just purchased her business and had no one else to run it. She was afraid of losing everything without being able to work. Do to her many years of training and good muscle strength, they only had to scrap out the area to repair it, but she has had years of dealing with back pain. Her sciatica nerve was also affected.

This started her down this long agonizing road of CF/ FM. I think she could tell you better than I how much she has had days she just wanted to end her suffering and find the Lord so she could ask why; why would he allow anyone to suffer so long and so hard. She has expressed this to me many times. I understand her thinking because I myself have been where she has been. I'm sure many others have also had these same thoughts. She has no doubt had many drugs. She developed a severe B-12 deficiency like I did. She had many tests and they couldn't tell her what was wrong. When I shared my symptoms with my physician, he knew right away what the problem was and put me on B-12 injections right away. I of course shared this with her and when they did the proper test found that indeed she was B-12 deficient. I'm sure she also was dealing with leaky gut and food intolerances. She has also had many of the same symptoms I have suffered from over the years. She is now getting treatments for cancer that they can't find but say is somewhere in her body. I have read that many people dealing with CF/FM will go on to develop cancer. I believe this is because of their inability to methylate toxins and the huge amount of exposures we all have had to toxic substances.

I have read that just one nutritional deficiency can cause disease in the body. Unfortunately our modern medical model doesn't teach regular M.D.'s to look for nutrient deficiencies. This is where functional medicine really shines and the reason I believe every doctor needs to be trained in this modality.

I've had days I just prayed the Lord would shorten my days on this earth so my misery would end. No one can know how much pain another person is in by looking at them. This much I know for a fact; the overwhelming fatigue that limits your life activities when you are a very active person before becoming disabled is also very frustrating. Although I suffered fatigue for years after being exposed on the soldering job, I pushed through the fatigue and remained active, until I became totally debilitated with the shoulder injury.

THE LORD'S HAND ON MY LIFE

I'm sure that most people with as many neuro-toxins and chemical exposures that I have had along with tragic life events would have succumbed to cancer or something by now. That is how I know the Lord has had his hand on my life and a good reason for why I'm still here and writing this book. Maybe it is that little prayer that I would help as many people as I could when I found some answers that has kept me here. Of course my path of avoiding drugs and relying on whole live foods, along with essential oils and herbs has no doubt also kept me going.

I have been privileged to find some of the best doctor's research that I know is available. My own test results and experiences confirm that everything they are saying is true and the cause of my health challenges. I was diagnosed with leaky gut syndrome by an osteopath who did the first chelations to get rid of fatigue and the calcium in the shoulder joint. He explained to me how having leaky gut can cause problems in the Krebs energy cycle. This is basically how sugars and amino acids enter the cells and are then converted to ATP for energy. He said the leaky gut could have come from the many impurities in the anti-inflammatory I was given for the shoulder injury. The long term disability carrier claimed I had celiac disease that caused my problems. I have had several tests for celiac since and they have all been negative. I did have high titer to gliadin when I had the leaky gut. They now know that you can have an intolerance to gluten without celiac and there are new tests for this, but when you have leaky gut, you can have an immune system reaction to anything and everything your eating depending on the severity of the problem. (See my articles on gluten intolerance and leaky gut) I had a number of the Elisa assay tests and they always showed different sensitivities to different foods.

I decided to turn my blog into a book so more people who need the access to this research could find it. I have had 16 years of searching and I believe this information is needed not only by those dealing with chronic fatigue/fibromyalgia, but anyone dealing with a chronic health condition.

NUTRITIONAL DEFICIENCIES

We have an epidemic of magnesium, iodine and selenium deficiencies because they have been depleted from the soil our food is produced on. Dr. Brownstein says that the bromide added to baked goods can block the iodine receptors. He also states the fluoride and chlorine in our water is an iodine blocker. Iodine is one nutrient that can help protect people from radiation fallout. A byproduct of chlorine in the processing of cotton is the production of dioxin. Dioxin is one of the most toxic carcinogens known to mankind. Can you think of some personal care products that might then contain dioxin?

One of the most intriguing things I found is that we all build antibodies to foods we eat. It only becomes a problem when we develop what is known as leaky gut syndrome and too many undigested proteins are absorbed through the intestinal tract causing an immune system reaction. Of course the first problem is poor digestion. Something, possibly a chemical or drug damages the pancreas and the pancreas no longer produces enough enzyme to break down a protein. In my case I didn't produce enough amylase so I wasn't breaking down carbohydrates. This showed up as high pyrovates in a blood test. No doubt all the muscle relaxers, anti-inflammatories and anti-biotics I had been prescribed contributed to this problem along with the heavy metal exposures.

The immune system sees any foreign protein in the blood as antigens. An antigen is a foreign invader. The immune system then mounts a response to deal with this problem. In this process the antibodies created send off a little charge when they encounter an antigen. This process can also damage delicate blood vessel linings. The immune system sees this damage to the blood vessels as something it has to repair. The immune system builds fibrin to go and patch this damage. Once fibrin is laid down, cholesterol and calcium build up causing plague to form. We now are on our way to developing heart disease. They know that one of the upper respiratory infections is notorious for this problem. What then is the result of introducing foreign DNA and other immune stimulants in vaccines? I believe there needs to be better research into this area of science.

Deficiencies or low levels of tyrosine may lead to iron deficiency. It also can lead to impaired metabolism of the amino acids methionine and taurine and have been linked to allergies and auto-immune disorders. Tyrosine is also necessary to produce serotonin and other neuro-transmitters. The doctor says he has done several tests and my iron levels are always perfect but I'm still anemic. This could be explained since lead interferes with hem synthesis in the blood.

It is obvious that we need a lot of anti-oxidants to protect us from the many toxins in our environment. We also need to keep the detox pathways working strong. One researcher stated that it is the reduced glutathione that causes accumulation of metals and toxins. I believe the metals and toxins burn the glutathione and other nutrients and prevent the proper detoxification process. The body was designed to produce glutathione, but with the many toxic substances we are being exposed to it is no wonder the body can't keep up with building enough glutathione to clear all these toxins from our bodies. Dr. Gary Gordon, is one physician who stated that, "we have 1,000 times the amount of lead in our bones than we had just 700 years ago." He should know since he has done tests for metals many times himself.

Nattokinase which is a soy based enzyme can be taken to break down fibrin. However if the blood is dealing with metals you may need higher doses of this enzyme to deal with the fibrin. I have learned that aluminum and magnesium when found together will cause the blood to become thick and form small mico-clots. This can lead to heart attack and stroke. I have taken the nattokinase and it does seem to help some of the muscle pain in fibromyalgia. I believe the reason for this is that it helps to clear out the small blood vessels. This allows more oxygen to flow to the tissues.

I recently read the opinion of one physician who said that toxins are a major cause for all illnesses. I believe this since it is oxidative stress (free radical species) that causes free radicals which can damage the DNA.

He stated that toxins also interfere with cell receptors that carry glucose to your muscles and fat cells. They can also limit your cells ability to use insulin. When your cells can't use glucose it causes a rise in blood sugars. Blood sugars are like glass scrapping the inside of the blood vessels. They know that natural sugars from foods are more easily used by the cells than cane sugar or high fructose corn syrup. I use natural fruits and nuts for snacks. It really isn't so hard to eat healthy if you follow a few simple rules. To eat a live food diet, just purchase food from the perimeter of your grocery store. This is where you will find the fruits and vegetables that provide the enzymes that help repair the body daily.

HELPFUL DIETARY TIPS

I heard a physician state that table salt is damaging to the blood vessel linings. He recommends you use sea salt instead. I have also read that table salt may contain aluminum and other toxins. With our oceans becoming polluted, this is another thing to be concerned about. Sometimes you just have to use your best judgment and hope for the best result.

If you avoid all processed foods your health will really thank you for it. Most processed foods contain trans fats or hydrogenated oils which are made from synthetic oils. I read that people who consume the most trans fats have the highest levels of pain as they get older. They passed a law to take some of these fats out of processed foods but it is wise to read the labels. I always look for baked potato chips because these products are not usually processed with trans fats.

The phosphates in pop will deplete the body of calcium. And there are over a hundred body processes that are dependent on calcium. Of course the extremely high content of sugar is contributing to our epidemic of obesity in this country. I just read that drinking one pop a day will put on 10 lbs of body weight per year. I think it would be higher for me. I don't do well with high amounts of sugar.

We can get a lot of calcium from vegetables, it isn't just found in milk products! Beans and greens are high in calcium. Phosphates can also build up in the muscle tissue of anyone dealing with FM because the cells can't get rid of it. This just leads to more pain so be sure you are not causing yourself more problems by indulging too much! I make an ice cream float with root beer on rare occasions, the dairy in the ice cream might offset some of the problem with phosphates.

HELPFUL TESTS

I had the privilege of having my blood looked at under the microscope; this can tell you what is going on in the blood. I don't know why this isn't the first thing a doctor looks at when they want to know how the body is actually functioning. You can see if there is fibrin or if there is a high level of free radical damage going on. You can also see if the blood cells are clumping together or if they are free floating. You will see if there are crystals which would indicate poor digestion of fats. This might be a good sign if you are chelating. Some crystals might indicate that you have high uric acid in excess. They may also get an idea if you are dealing with high amounts of sugars in the blood or anemia. If the blood looks light in the middle of the cell, you may not be processing sugars well. If the digestion is poor mico particles might be present. Yeasts or fungus might show up as white circles in serum. Undigested foods might show up as darkened areas. You might even see evidence of heavy metal damage. Holistic doctors and chiropractors are the only physicians I know that might use this as a diagnostic tool. I wonder why it isn't part of every physician's office. I think it could be a very valuable tool.

I came across a good chart from a group of physicians in California who treat CF/FM. I spoke with one of these physicians and he said he had heavy metal problems himself. This is why he got into chelation therapy as a protocol to help his patients. You can find them on the internet under the Holtorf medical clinic in California.

They came up with an excellent chart that explains how the process of developing these conditions can occur. At the top of his chart is physical stressor which leads to sleep disorder, G.I. impairment, nutrient deficiencies, mitochondrial damage, auto-immmunity, immune dysfunction, reactivated latent infections, and the underlying problem is environmental toxins. Some people however may produce more enzymes to deal with toxins; it might be those who have had the least exposures to deplete the glutathione.

I believe they have a clear picture of what causes chronic fatigue/fibromyalgia and many chronic undiagnosed illnesses. He said I wouldn't get well until I got rid of the metals. I also had a physician who did a challenge for me who said he and his wife were both ill with these illnesses and this lead him into learning about chelation therapy and holistic health. They also both had high levels of metals. This illness knows no boundaries; it is affecting every segment of society. I believe that the deficiencies of nutrients in the food chain along with an overload of environmental toxins is causing the health care crisis that we see going on around us today. My physician says he has 30 year olds that can't do anything. I also had a retired nurse from church say when she was in physical therapy there were young people in there that were like 90 year olds and could barely move.

I think as you read through the chapters in this book you will see a clear outline of all the body systems that are affected by these problems. There is a urine test called the IAG test that looks for a metabolite of tryptophan. Many researchers believe that when this is present it would indicate a "leaky gut syndrome" there is still debate over this issue; it has been found in autism and chronic fatigue patients. The Elisa assay will look for antibodies being produced toward food proteins indicating a leaky gut.

LEADING RESEARCHERS

As Dr. Rigden (named leading researcher on CF/FM) stated in a recent article "leaky gut syndrome" and toxic heavy metals along with drugs like NSAIDs, cortisone, and antibiotics, stress, parasites, yeast, and viral infections are all contributors to the development of these syndromes, of course having a direct exposure to metals is a definite cause to disease.

Most of the immune system does its work through the pyres patches along the intestinal tract. These patches are responsible for producing IGA antibodies that fight off bacteria and viruses. When the intestinal tract becomes inflamed these antibodies can become damaged and unable to do their job. This leaves a person vulnerable for infections.

Being under stress can also cause a drop in the production of these antibodies. This is probably why we catch more colds and flu when we are stressed. I have found Echinacea to be helpful. If you have a very active immune system you might be cautious in taking this herb. Astragalus is another herb which has been used in China to boost the immune system.

TRAGIC SITUATIONS

One of the most tragic cases that I have come across of someone dealing with CF/FM was a clinic physician who became totally disabled. She was cut off from her long term disability insurance at the two year own occupation limit. She tried to fight this but found that she was getting nowhere. When she became aware that many others were dealing with this same issue she started to gather evidence of these cases. She tried to get a lawyer to help her but seem to get a run around. Then she tried to represent herself. She finally found a lawyer who said he would start a class action for her.

I don't know why this class action did not go forward. I would learn later that she developed M.S. and a brain tumor along with the diagnosis of CF/FM. When she finally got before a judge they agreed to give her two years for depression and nothing on the other diagnosis. I couldn't believe this. She had 5 doctors saying she was permanently disabled. I spoke with her previous lawyer and he made the comment to me, "be careful or you might end up like Judy Doc (as she was affectionately known)." I asked what happened to her and he said he didn't want to discuss her case. He said the more noise you make the more determined they are not to help you. She went on Medicaid since she was on so many drugs that were expensive and Medicare would not cover all of them. She had to take in a roommate to help her meet her expenses. She had a long term disability policy that should have paid her 90% of her pay for as long as she was disabled. You may think you are safe if you have a disability policy but find out you can't collect past the two year own occupation limit these companies have been allowed to change their policies to without telling the clients their policies had been changed.

I just read on the Lawyers And Settlements site that many cases that were ordered to be compensated by one insurer are still being denied their monies. You can learn more about this by visiting their website.

I still can't believe anyone with any moral fiber could treat a human being like Judy Doc was treated. The only thing I can think of is that they wanted to set and example for anyone else who might try to fight the broken system. Her case is very tragic because she ended her own plight. I wonder how many other victims of the system are out there. I do know this, there will be many more if we don't take a stand to make them enforce the laws that are on the books and dismiss any judge that steps outside the boundaries of the law. We have people who are interpreting the law instead of enforcing the law. This sentiment was recently expressed during the republican debates. Our politicians are aware that people have lost their rights in many situations. One politician stated, "people have lost their worker's rights and their human rights." Judy shared with me that she thought she had been followed and was run off the road. Social security recognizes depression as a disabling disorder; then why isn't the long term disability carriers ordered to also compensate this for as long as the person is disabled?

This is not an isolated case. There have been several class actions against long term disability insurers. It seems that many are being forced to sue to insure their rights but the people who cannot afford lawyers and court fees are losing their rights. This has to change to restore fairness and equity to working people. You might think you are secure because you pay for long term disability insurance, but you may find it impossible to collect when you most need it, unless of course you can afford the high expense of good lawyers and court fees. I was told this could run in the tens of thousands of dollars.

I recently learned of a case of CF/FM where the person had high ammonia levels. I have read that even a slightly elevated level of ammonia in the blood can lead to brain damage. She recently had her colon removed. I asked what happened; she had been on many pain meds for a chronic condition. This can lead to auto-intoxication through the colon walls according to Dr. Gilbere. She had her insurance cancelled before going in for surgery; this meant a reduction of around $500.00 per month for her family. I find it ironic that the people who are suppose to insure our rights are enforced never have to worry about losing their health, they have voted themselves permanent health insurance, yet they are failing the American people by not making these companies do what is right.

OUR MORAL OBLIGATION

One Sunday the sermon was on making your life a life that really counts. The minister said we need to focus on what we can do to make life better not only for ourselves but for others. He also said we need to find something that we are willing to give our lives for and be willing to lay our lives down for and fight for if necessary. Too many people in the "me" generation have been living life for themselves not caring what happened in the world. I think too many people have been asleep while evil has been running the planet!

Many won't even watch the news because it might disturb them and they don't think they can do anything about what is going on anyway. Well wake up people Ron Paul just said American is gone it doesn't exist anymore. So when these "me" people lose everything they have worked hard for the wake up call might be blaring! Like President Obama stated when he was running for election, "no one should lose everything they have because they became disabled." He said he was going to try and right this injustice that had been going on for too long.

Our forefathers founded this nation on Christian principals, yet a small group of non-believers claims discrimination and the law shifts to accommodate them. Christians need to wake up and speak up for their rights! This is what our forefathers meant for this great nation when they drew up the declaration of independence. Does anyone remember their history? Patrick Henry was probably one of the greatest patriots when he said, "give me liberty or give me death." Our liberties and our rights have been slowly eaten away.

If we don't wake up we will look around and not be able to recognize this nation. Everyone seems to be living in a state of fear. When you fear your own government you need a wake up call. Now they want to pass a law that they can label anyone a threat to the nation without due process of the law. What are we coming to? This is the kind of thing that goes on in dictatorships. Shame on those who voted for this! They may themselves become a victim someday. Dictators after all have targeted those at the top as well as those in society in their own countries.

We have been going to war in the name of securing other peoples freedoms while slowly losing those freedoms here at home. I believe we have a right to freedom of speech that is what this nation was founded on. If that is ever taken away then we might as well be living under communism and can no longer call ourselves a democracy. We need to wake up and see the e-v-i-l going on all around us!

I recently read a book by senator Dement and he had a lot to say about what is going on in Washington. He has taken a hard stand and is trying to do what is right. Others who at first gave him opposition are now lining up with him. Sometimes it just takes one brave soul to start a movement. One small voice can change a nation. I hope he keeps up the good work! I am tired of politics as usual. We need people who keep their campaign promises to the people of this great nation.

Many senators are getting pressured to pass legislation they haven't even had time to read. Unbelievable but true. We could wake up one morning to being owned by some other entity. Our future as a nation is at stake. I had one young person say, "so maybe that wouldn't be so bad." I wanted to say do you remember the names Stalin and Hitler? Evil flourishes when good men and women do nothing.

Let us not be part of letting evil flourish lets be part of making this a better world for our children and our grandchildren!

What scares me the most is that our children seem to have the attitude that no one can do anything? We have had to fight to preserve liberty for others around the world but we seem to shrink back in fear to defend our own rights and freedoms. Its time to take a stand for what is right! We have the God given right to take care of our minds and bodies as we see fit. The Bible even states "physician heal thyself."

Elaine Marie Graham

WHAT IS GOING ON IN HEALTHCARE

It makes me ill when people on Medicaid say they have to take the medicines they tell them to take or they might lose their healthcare. Every person should have the right to choose what medicines and what supplements they feel best meets the needs of their body. They go so far as to say they test their blood to make sure they are taking certain medications. I find this hard to believe but I have heard this! I do believe we need to stop the pre-existing exemptions for all health issues. No one should be excluded from health care because they changed jobs or became ill. None of our senators ever have to worry about pre-existing exemptions in their health care.

No one knows your body like you do and no one should have the right to dictate what you will or won't take, especially if what your taking is causing a nasty side affect. Surely this needs to change. I would have been dead a long time ago if I listened to what the doctors told me to do every time. People with FM can not tolerate many medications. They do much better with natural herbs and supplements. This is why they need a physician that is not only an M.D. but has training in holistic or functional medicine.

I believe drugs should be used as a last resort not the first course of treatment. Everyone's metabolism and body works differently, that is why one drug may help one person and be toxic to another. Someday they may be able to test you to see what is compatible with your system before they prescribe treatment, but for now we need to be vigilant against side affects. I am only aware of toxic affects from natural herbs when a person over consumed them for some reason or mixes them with medications that have interactions.

LET FOOD BE YOUR MEDICINE

Holistic or functional medicine is not something new. People used herbs and foods as medicine for centuries before there were pharmaceutical companies. Most people had their own herb gardens. My grandparents used dandelion roots and ginseng. They knew these contained a lot of great medicinal properties. They hunted for the ginseng because it was a very valuable commodity.

My mother shared with me that when she was growing up her mother gave her some dandelion greens and a dose of cod liver oil in the spring and fall. This helps purge the intestines of any unfriendly visitors.

We must also be vigilant to eat a healthy diet. If we could avoid exposures to toxic substances whenever possible it would really help. I believe the world is finally waking up to these same issues but it will take vigilance to keep in place laws that will protect the public from the dangers lurking in our personal and health care products. I think it would be wise to follow Europe's lead and make laws that require something be found safe before it is put in to use by the consumer.

We must be vigilant to support the rights of injured workers and to make sure the laws that are already in place are honored. Those dealing with long term disability insurance should not have to worry about losing this insurance for as long as they are disabled. Too many people have been denied their rights.

WHERE TO BEGIN?

Functional medicine is saying you must first address the food intolerances, remove the toxins from the system to the degree possible, heal the leaky gut and eat a healthy diet to maintain your health and to regain it if you have already lost it. Sometimes the damage is beyond repair and you have to learn to live with it, as seen in so many cases of fibromyalgia because people did not get the care they needed.

"Circulating immune complexes happen because you have proteins in the blood from the leaky gut," according to Dr. Gary Gordon. He suffered from poor methylation and had to close his medical practice at age 29. He has done much research into the affects of heavy metals and has come up with his own 5 step program to achieve and maintain health. He also recently stated in a live video that our lead levels were high before they took lead out of gasoline in the early 80's. He should know since he was involved with the developing of these laboratory tests for heavy metal exposures.

Many who have fallen ill have not had the financial help to address their issues from a holistic approach. If you look at Dr. Tietelbaum's approach for example, it requires a lot of supplementation. Anyone who has been ill for a while could easily become overwhelmed by the emotional and financial pressures of being ill. When you can't work or are forced on disability you surely don't have all the funds needed for all the supplements that have been suggested. I'm sure there are those who suffer from post traumatic stress from years of being ill and not getting the care they needed.

It is my experience that if the toxic issues are not addressed, as Dr. Cheney said they need to be, you will also not get well. It has been my experience that exposure to toxic metals can insight your immune system for years. The fact that no one looked for this for years has no doubt contributed to my still experiencing problems in restoring my own health. It is essential that our doctors get educated regarding the conditions of CF/FM and there contributing factors. I would recommend that anyone dealing with any health issue seek out a holistic or functional medicine physician. They look for the root of the problem, they don't just treat the symptoms of the problem.

Dr. Mark Hyman M.D. recently stated on facebook, "Chronic illness—whether physical or mental, dementia, depression, ADHD, autism, chronic fatigue, obesity disease, cancer and allergic and auto-immune diseases are all related to elevated levels of cytokines and system inflammation." "They can cause problems in every organ in every part of the body." This should impress upon the establishment just how vitally important it is to get our environmental exposures under control. They are after all breathing the same air and eating the same foods that we are.

RESEARCH ARTICLES ON CF/FM

While doing my research over the past sixteen years, I have been privileged to come across several very helpful articles especially if you're fighting for disability.

The first is a copy of a House of Representatives bill regarding fibromyalgia that was done in June of 1999. This bill recognizes the severity of this problem and some of the contributing factors which are stress, trauma, or possibly an infectious agent in susceptible people. Let us not forget that the top treating physician in the U.S., Dr. Paul Cheney said these people are loaded with all kinds of chemicals, pesticides and heavy metals and have to be detoxed before they will see improvement. I have a copy of his report.

The Fibromyalgia Network put out a report dated Jan. '92 that stated. "Four studies have said that fibromyalgia syndrome (FMS) can be as disabling as rheumatoid arthritis (RA). "One would think that based on these three studies alone, the disability issue on FMS was an open and closed case." "FMS subjects also experienced the same level of problems as RA individuals in areas of mobility, walking and bending, arm function, household tasks, social activities, exercise, fatigue, work, mood and health perceptions."

The Fibromyalgia Syndrome Political Case Statement Fibromyalgia Network 1/96 states, "Researchers have noted a significant overlap between FMS and Chronic Fatigue syndrome (CFS) and a majority of patients who meet the diagnostic criteria for FMS also meet the CDC criteria for CFS."

If you think you may have bacteria from the gut (mycoplasmas) they can be tested for. You might look up The Arthritis Research Institute in Gaithersburg, Md. 20877. Their phone number is 301-216-1231. Many people who develop leaky gut may be dealing with this issue. It was found that people with RA had mycoplasmas in their joints.

I highly suggest you get the book from "Wellness Resources" on the Leptin Diet it is called "Mastering Leptin" by Byron J. Richards, CCN with Mary Guignon Richards. He has a chapter on FM and he definitely understands it!!!!!!!!!!!

There has been a dysfunction of the neurotransmitters in the brain of people with CF/FM. It isn't just a state of depression. They are finding these neurotransmitters to be low. I believe this problem starts with inflammation. I recently read they are saying that depression starts with a pro-inflammatory state. My nurse practitioner stated, "If you have inflammation in the gut you will have it all over the body." When you read my article on tests for leaky gut, you will see that the tryptophan is being lost in the urine. This neurotransmitter is necessary to produce serotonin and serotonin is necessary to produce melatonin. I believe it is inflammation that is the precursor for developing the leaky gut. This might be due to trauma and stress hormones, chemicals (drugs), heavy metal exposures, bacteria's, yeasts or parasites. I remember reading an article on food allergies and their connection to allergies of the brain tissues. They know there is a direct correlation of the nervous system in the gut relaying impulses to the brain. I also just recently read they believe an auto-immune condition may be causing antibodies to destroy the serotonin in the gut.

Neurotransmitters are what the brain uses to tell the body what to do. In Fibromyalgia there is an abnormal production of neurotransmitters such as serotonin, melatonin, norepinephrine, dopamine, and other chemicals which help control pain, mood, sleep and the immune system. Often there has been a trigger event, such as an accident. What does this have to do with developing these problems. Look at what the leading researcher says, "anti-biotics, cortisone, and anti-inflammatories all can lead to leaky gut syndrome," which also causes poor absorption of nutrients and these are readily administered to injured patients. He also states heavy metals can lead to leaky gut as well. This obviously explains the genesis of my problems.

A study by the American College of Rheumatology in 1992 found that the impact of FMS on your life is as bad, or worse than RA.

In addition, several amino acids in the blood have also been found to be present in lower than normal concentrations, including, the amino acid precursor that makes serotonin in the brain. Both serotonin and norepinephrine are thought to play a major role in the modulation of pain, inadequate amounts of either chemical can increase a person's pain sensitivity.

A study of 30 pain-free controls and twenty-nine FMS patients identified the FMS patients from controls with an accuracy rate of 82% by 7 biochemical variables (plasma histidine, methionine, tryptophan, norepinephrine, isoleucine, and urinary dopamine).

Since most patients of CF/FM do not do well with drugs, you might want to consider trying 5-htp from the health food store to help elevate mood and serotonin. Many people say it helps lift their mood and improve sleep. Of course melatonin is also helpful on those sleepless nights when you know sleep won't come easy. There is also a product called "Replete Extra" which has L-tyrosine, 5-hydroxytrptophan, and folate acid which functional medical doctors sometimes use.

According to the Montague/Hooper Paper 1 st May 2001 cognitive behavioral therapy has been shown to be of no long-term benefit in the disorders of ME/CFS. I believe this is because it is a physiological problem and not a psychological one! I said I was depressed because I was in pain not that I had pain because I was depressed!!!!!!!!! And guess what, I was right!!!!!!!!!! Many who have had to suffer with these syndromes have emotional scars from all the sarcasm that has been thrown their way and from being told "it's all in your head". They are owed more than an apology. These people need support and understanding not ridicule from society.

Many of our soldiers have returned from Iraq and Afghanistan with these conditions. No doubt they have had many toxic exposures along with tremendous stress. Just go to a support meeting with someone and find out for yourself the horror of these conditions that these people are dealing with and you may change your outlook on the subject. Your feelings may change to those of outrage at the injustice many have had to deal with! You might even realize this could happen to anyone, everyone is at risk for developing these conditions today with the entire heavy load of chemicals we are exposed to and toxins in our environment. The leading visit to emergency rooms is now severe body wide muscle pain! No doubt many are dealing with leaky gut syndrome!

President Clinton made a statement when he was in office to the effect that if we did not get the pollution in our environment under control we might not survive as a species. Certainly all the natural disasters that we are experiencing may be directly related to the pollution in the atmosphere which has been depleting the ozone for years. Pictures of the poles surely expose the fact that our ice mantels are being rapidly depleted. I don't think anyone can deny that we are polluting our environment faster than nature is able to clean it up.

It is frightening to me that the polar bears are even showing toxins in their systems one wouldn't think would be there. I fear our problems will only keep being compounded unless we wake up and realize we don't have time to waste. We must act now to reverse this trend of pollution as usual. We need to be active in letting our representatives know that we have to act to stop the pollution of our coal burning plants that are spewing out tons of toxic waste in to our environment.

A young college student has invented a device which can be placed on exhaust systems of cars to cut down the carbon emissions. I wonder if they will allow this to be brought to market or will the special interests that want to produce electric cars win the day.

WHERE DOES ALL THE POLLUTION COME FROM

Coal powered electric plants create two-thirds of the nation's sulfur dioxide emissions, which cause the acid rain that kills trees and pollutes lakes. They also produce a quarter of the nitrogen oxides that make smog: about 35 percent of mercury, which contaminates fish and can cause brain damage in fetuses if eaten by pregnant women; and about 40 percent of carbon dioxide, which contributes to global warming, according to the Enviornmental Protection Agency.

Utility companies claim that taking steps to clean up their smoke stacks could raise electric bills and reduced energy supply. I think we need to take steps to help them with tax breaks or incentives to put scrubbers on these smoke stacks so that they can take steps to clean up the environment. These arguments have been going on since President Bush was in office, and still there haven't been any changes made! Studies have shown that children who live in cities where there is more air pollution suffer higher rates of asthma and other childhood diseases. I think the research is clear, we need to act now! We can no longer go about business as usual. Doctor Oz mentioned that he was concerned about all the aluminum in the chemtrails. We need to ask what and why there are chemtrails and what else are they dumping into our environment.

When I was having chelation therapy I had a conversation with a teacher and she said she observes these chemtrails when she takes her children out for recess. I observed them while visiting a friend in Az. She has been concerned for some time about this situation. I watched them lay down a tic-tac-toe grid and then the trails from the dumping spread out and came together to block out the sun. I observed this for three days. She says when this is happening there are more visits to the doctor's offices and that the physicians are concerned about it. We need to be asking what is going on. Even Dr. Oz said he was concerned about the amount of aluminum in our atmosphere from chemtrails. I learned from a video which was done by a naturopath that when you combine aluminum and magnesium it makes the blood form micro-clots. This could lead to stroke and heart attack.

They are finding toxins like uranium and plutonium in testing for metals. Where do these come from? They may come from natural terrain or they might be coming from use in missiles designed to destroy heavy metal armored vehicles in wars around the world. This could come from wind and rain currents. Of course oil spills and nuclear explosions have added to our current problems.

POLITICAL ACTION ON CF/FM

When I was first diagnosed with CF/FM we had an Indian doctor who was going about the country telling our doctors this was a somato "all in your head" form of disease.

It was very scary to me that someone could be responsible for these kinds of statements since I knew first hand the horrors of living with this problem. I have been actively trying to educate our politicians as to the real research that proves these people are dealing with a deregulated immune, endocrine and neurological system. The research has been overwhelming that this is true. There has been a lot of conjecture as to whether there is a genetic component in these conditions. I believe if you are dealing with leaky gut syndrome you can develop intolerances to gluten, dairy and many other foods but the research indicates this is an acquired condition and not a genetic one. I would have to totally agree with this. I had no pain before developing the leaky gut after my injury and drugs. I believe if something is truly genetic you would be dealing with it at birth, not years later, as most genetic diseases are obvious at birth. I said to my physician I didn't think I had a methylation problem before my exposures to the lead soldering job; it was after this exposure that I had the problem with fatigue. He agreed with me and said he didn't think I had the problem before that either.

See the Montague/Hooper Paper from 2001. This report indicates that an enzyme which is responsible for taking out viruses is damaged. They indicate this can happen due to toxins in the body. They state in the Montague/Hooper Paper that "the growing body of scientific literature clearly shows that there are profound disturbances of and damage to the neuro-endocrine-immune systems which must be understood as inter-connected systems that share many common messenger molecules". They also state that drug therapy in these patients is often precluded by serious adverse reactions. I believe this is due to the hyper-permeable state of the intestinal tract. They also state that environmental influences which worldwide researchers are investigating include the frequent pairing of CFS with food and chemical sensitivities.

There are a series of enzyme reactions which go on inside white blood cells when they perceive themselves to be challenged by a virus or some toxic exposure.

They suggest that the inability to tolerate physical activity is due to abnormal oxidative metabolism. This they say might be linked to defective interferon responses.

We now know that the mitochondria which is the power house within the cells is damaged and cannot produce energy from the amino acids and glucose that is introduced to the cells.

Researchers worldwide are now looking at the frequent pairing of CFS with food and chemical sensitivities. Dr. Howard Umovitz from the Chronic Illness Research Foundation at Berkeley, California, whose work has been published in the Journal of American Society for Microbiology and in Clinical Microbiology Reviews; has demonstrated a fundamental breakthrough linking toxic exposure with chronic diseases such as ME/CFS and other auto-immune disorders. He suggests that the huge increase in chemical usage is chronically stimulating the immune system.

Urinary creatine test at the British Society of Rheumatologists Conference in Edinburgh, April 2001, evidence was presented which showed that patients with ME/CFS are excreting in their urine significant levels of creatine and other muscle related metabolites including choline and glycine. This they said may represent evidence of on-going muscle damage in ME/CFS. Creatine has previously been shown to be a sensitive marker of muscle inflammation.

It has been suggested that the measurement of the CD4-CD8 ratio be measured. Tests should also include ANAs (antinuclear antibodies), IgGs, including IgE, CiCs (circulating immune complexes) IL2:IL4 (interleukin 2 and 4) and Th1-Th2 response and mitogen stimulation tests. Also tests for thyroid antibodies should be done.

They state that "psychiatric disorder is not a core aspect of CFS and that this is a strong argument against CFS being a psychosomatic or functional somatic disorder."

There is evidence of a degenerative process of the muscle tissue in CFS patients, as typically occurs in mitochondrial myopathies. This may contribute to muscle fatigability and it supports an organic origin for CFS.

Latent viruses may activate a coagulation of the blood. The blood can also form clots when you are exposed to heavy metals especially aluminum and magnesium. This is why I believe Nattokinase soy based enzyme is so important. Dr. Oz stated on his show that if you take this you won't have to worry about heart attack or stroke.

Our bodies have a system in place to handle toxins. It does not however know how to handle all the new toxins in our environment. Therefore they may accumulate to harmful quantities or be converted to odd unknown substances that can interfere with metabolism. This results in cancers and birth defects.

There are a number of helpful therapies to help the body rid itself of toxins. These include fasting (spoken of in the bible, Epsom salts baths, hydrotherapy, diet and nutrition, herbs, chelation, and exercise. The infrared sauna is also used in Europe to help release toxins from the tissues. The master lemon cleanse is also very helpful to help raise the bodies ph levels.

One supplement that is becoming popular is glutathione. Glutathione is what the body uses to rid itself of toxins. It is produced in the liver and blood. Some people dealing with metals that are struggling with the methylation system may need to take reduced glutathione in order to boost their elimination of toxins. I have read that most glutathione produces on the market will be destroyed by the digestive enzymes in the stomach.

I tried a product called Advanced Methyl Caps by Complementary prescriptions. Unfortunately this seemed to make my pain much worse. This was before I had a study done by Genova Diagnostics to look at the methylation pathways. I am now trying a different approach. I am taking Dr. Rudy Cartwrights Essentials formula that has reduced glutathione in it. I could feel my pain level come down the first week. I am also taking B-12, B-6 zink, flax and evening primrose and several other nutrients. A metyl form of folic acid is essential to assist the detox pathways.

I recently came across an article that indicated mercury potentiates the deleterious effects or organophosphates on neurotransmitters. If this is true it is more important than ever to try and eat organic foods and avoid pesticides.

It has also been said that mercury toxicity is associated with malfunction of ACH receptors. It also causes apoptosis of cells. Mercury blocks receptors for acetylcholine and other neuro-transmitters by immune complexes of mercury and its antibody. No wonder it can cause neuro-endocrine problems.

Tests can be done to determine if you have a genetic tendency for gluten intolerance. This can be done by a swab of the mucosa lining of the mouth. Some people may have an intolerance to dairy in which you can produce the GAD's antibody. The GAD's antibody is an antibody produced by the immune system that attacks proteins of dairy. There may be a genetic tendency to be more reactive to certain foods or chemicals. Of course developing the leaky gut also leads to food protein reactions.

In the process of attacking these antigens; if they get into the system, much destruction can be done. They are finding that people with M.S. should not eat gluten. See Dr. Rudy Cartwright for more information on this. He has a formula for people suffering with M.S. It has catalase, (reduced) glutathione, quercitin, hesperiden, catechin & acetylcysteine, also niacin. I have used this and have not gotten the niacin flush which I would normally get with a niacin supplement. You can find Dr. Cartwright on the internet if you do a search. I have also read that gluten antibodies can cause Hashimoto's thyroid disorders. One interesting article on reversing oxidative stress suggested that once oxidative stress is reversed, this condition may reverse itself.

If your digestion is complete and you are producing enough digestive enzymes like pancreatin, lipase, amylase your immune system should not react to proteins which are consumed. However if you develop leaky gut or an intolerance to a protein it can set off an immune system reaction. See my articles on leaky gut for more information on this. You will have to heal the leaky gut to allow the immune system to return to a normal state. You may also have to rid your system of the heavy burden of toxic chemicals and metals.

My doctor told me to eat a salad every day. Greens have lots of folic acid which is healing to the gut. Luckily I love salad! I was also advised to use digestive enzymes which can help bring the pain levels down if you're dealing with reactions to foods or leaky gut syndrome. A good formula will have at least 10,000 IU (international units) of protease in it along with the amylase and lipase. Remember Dr. Paul Cheney cautioned that these people are dealing with an overload of chemicals, pesticides and heavy metals. He says you have to detox them first to get results. See the articles on heavy metals!

I have also used the "Master Lemon Cleanse" which is the fastest way to calm down an over-active immune system and cleanse the system of toxins. This is simple. You just use 2-3 Tablespoons of maple syrup in a glass of 6-8 ounces of water with 1/2 lemon and a pinch of cayenne. This can be taken up to 12 times in an 8 hr. period. I usually only get 5-6 glasses down. Two days on this cleanse without food is the easiest way to fast and you still get your vitamins and minerals you need. The best juice fast for inflammation I've found is golden delicious apples, 1/2 inch of Ginger and carrots. This got my son off the couch in two days when he was down with pancreatitis. Dr. Oz said take ginger pills every day if you have joint pain. Ginger helps fight cancers and inflammation. You may also want to try curcumin which has been shown to fight cancer, lower cholesterol and tryglicerides and fight inflammation. Dr. Oz also demonstrated that Vitamin D is like a pacman eating up cancer cells. They recommend you take curcumin with a little warm olive oil so it is absorbed better. I would think taking it with a meal would also help.

The Chronic Fatigue Association is now publishing research from around the world. They also have a site on which you can leave comments, so you'll want to check this out. More people need to speak out so fewer people have to deal with this in the future. The Bible says the greatest thing a person can do with their life is to help someone else with their health but some people are resistant to help. I'm sure many of you have family members like this! Don't give up—just keep sharing information something you say may help.

The Montague Hooper Paper from 2001 states:

"The endocrine system is uniquely disrupted in ME/CFS. A key feature is the demonstrated defect in HPA axis function (55.56) and patients are severely limited by the loss of dynamic hormone responses." "There is an abnormality of adrenal function and CT scans have shown that both the right and left adrenal glands are reduced by 50% when compared with controls.

The adrenals are responsible for many body functions. The most important may be that they provide the body with powerful stress hormone cortisol. Cortisol helps dial down pain levels, sharpens your mind, heightens mood, gives extra energy on demand, suppresses allergies, influences sleep cycle! However too much cortisol production can become toxic to the body. Dr. Cheney stated that you can lose control over the adrenals if the hypothalamus adrenal axis is off for too long.

No wonder people are suffering from fatigue, memory problems, sleep disturbance, need for daytime naps, weight gain especially belly fat! The adrenals are exhausted! The adrenals also stimulate the liver to produce glycogen which is stored over night and released to keep you from going into a low blood sugar and coma. The adrenals regulate blood pressure by secreting adrenaline! They also produce DHEA and testosterone which can be low in CF/FM.

Adrenals help fight fatigue, insomnia, infections, asthma, obesity and even thyroid problems. Too much cortisol is like searing acid which can eat away at delicate body tissues. You can also develop a metabolic weight loss syndrome when the adrenals are over producing adrenaline or cortisol. I once read that the reason people who get in severe sudden accidents actually die is from the rush of stress hormones to the gut that cause the gut to leak and the whole body becomes filed with sepsis. They then go into shock and coma. I found this interesting. Then is it any wonder that when we have a trauma or prolonged stress and continually have these same hormones going to the gut that this tissue becomes weak and hyper-permeable?

Long term stress can also run down the adrenal function and the adrenals become exhausted from wear and tear. Weight gain around the thighs or stomach can indicate the adrenals are sluggish!

WELLNESS RESOURCES

The Wellness Resources has a couple products I think work well when you are under stress. The first one is "stress helper". This product contains (Pantethine, acetyl-l-carnitine, and carnosine) provide energy producing cofactors to help the body cope with the demands of stress. They also help the body settle back into a more normal baseline of energy production once the stress is over, helping to avert wear and tear. Pantethine also improves mental clarity and supports adrenal function. Pantethine makes Coenzyme A (CoA) a pivotal nutrient in at least 70 energy-related metabolic pathways, including those that make adrenal hormones. You may take 300-1,800 mg of pantethine to help offset stress demands and support adrenal health.

Dr. Paul Cheney stated that you may detoxify these patients (CF/FM) but they may be left with defects in dynamic hypothalamic control, particularly of the dynamic hormones, cortisol and growth hormone. I was told by a physician who had CF/FM herself if you have low thyroid and adrenal function and it isn't addressed through intervention you can be left with permanent damage in the tissues. What Dr. Cheney says confirms this for me.

LOW NEUROTRANSMITTERS IN CF/FM

There has been a dysfunction of the neurotransmitters in the brain of people with CF/FM. It isn't just a state of depression

Neurotransmitters are what the brain uses to tell the body what to do. In Fibromyalgia there is an abnormal production of neurotransmitters such as serotonin, melatonin, norepinephrine, dopamine, and other chemicals which help control pain, mood, sleep and the immune system. Often there has been a trigger event, such as an accident. What does this have to do with developing these problems? Look at what Dr. Scott Rigden named the leading researcher of the year a couple years ago said—anti-biotics, cortisone, and anti-inflammatories along with heavy metals can lead to leaky gut syndrome which also causes poor absorption of nutrients and these drugs are readily administered to injured patients.

A study by the American College of Rheumatology in 1992 found that the impact of FMS on your life is as bad, as or worse than RA.

In addition, several amino acids in the blood have also been found to be present in lower than normal concentrations, including, the amino acid precursor that makes serotonin in the brain. Both serotonin and norepinephrine are thought to play a major role in the modulation of pain—inadequate amounts of either chemical can increase a person's pain sensitivity.

A study of 30 pain-free controls and twenty-nine FMS patients identified the FMS patients from controls with an accuracy rate of 82% by 7 biochemical variables (plasma histidine, methionine, tryptophan, norepinephrine, isoleucine, and urinary dopamine).

Since most patients of CF/FM do not do well with drugs, you might want to consider trying 5-htp from the health food store to help elevate mood and serotonin. Many people say it helps lift their mood and improve sleep. Of course melatonin is also helpful on those sleepless nights.

According to the Montague/Hooper Paper 1 st May 2001 cognitive behavioural therapy has been shown to be of no long-term benefit in the disorders of ME/CFS. I believe this is because it is a physiological problem and not a psychological one! I said I was depressed because I was in pain not that I had pain because I was depressed!!!!!!!!! And guess what I was right!!!!!!!!!! Many who have had to suffer with these syndromes have emotional scars from all the sarcasm that has been thrown their way. These people need support and understanding not ridicule from society. Just go to a support group meeting with someone and find out for yourself the horror of these conditions that these people are dealing with and you may be ashamed of the thoughts you have had toward these people. Your feelings may change to those of outrage at the injustice many have had to deal with! You might even realize this could happen to anyone, everyone is at risk for developing these conditions today with the entire heavy load of chemicals we are exposed to and toxins in our environment.

DIET AND CHRONIC FATIGUE/FIBROMYALGIA

It has been found that a whole live foods diet is the best diet for the conditions of chronic fatigue/fibromyalgia. I believe the reason for this is simple. It is the live fruits and vegetables that are full of enzymes. Enzymes are used by the body to repair and rebuild body organs and tissues. Avoiding processed foods high in trans fats is also very helpful.

Epidemiological evidence exists that indicate there is a correlation between increased dietary intake of anti-oxidants and a lower incidence of morbidity and mortality. This isn't surprising since it is free radical damage that leads to inflammation within the body. Doctors are now attributing inflammation to most all diseases.

The curcumin (tumeric) has been found to reduce blood cholesterol, prevent low-density lipoprotein oxidation, inhibit platelet aggregation, thrombosis and myocardial infarction, suppresses symptoms assoc. with type II diabetes. R.A. M.S. and Alzheimer disease, inhibits HIV replication, suppresses tumor formation, enhances wound healing, protects liver injury, increases bile secretion, protects against cataract formation, and protects against pulmonary toxicity and fibrosis.

Curcumin is a favorite of M.D. Anderson Cancer Center according to my latest readings. Here is what they say—curcumin directly damages the DNA of colon cancer cells, repairs damage to DNA of cells damaged by arsenic poisoning. There are high levels of arsenic in our soil so it may also be found in water and food supplies.

CANDIDA

Candida has been associated with "leaky gut syndrome" by holistic physicians and integrative medicine physicians.

Candida may get out of control when we are treated with anti-biotics which kill off the beneficial flora. After taking a round of anti-biotics it is wise to supplement the gut flora with the beneficial flora lactobacillus, acidophilus and bifidus. There are many formulas on the market but your integrative physician may have one he would like to recommend.

You may need to go on a diet which eliminates sugar since candida are known to feed on candida.

There are many natural products you can use to help keep the candida in check while your on the candida diet. Apple cider vinegar, and coconut oil are effective along with garlic oil, grapefruit seed extract, and other natural anti-fungals.

Avoid alcohol as it produces acetaldehyde. Yogurt also contains some helpful probiotics. Digestive enzymes kill candida directly and are synergistic with antifungals. Papaine and bromelaine are also very helpful.

We used a product called Colostrum. Colostrum is the pre-milk taken from the cow after it has given birth. This has many beneficial properties especially specific antibodies that address bacterial and fungal issues. Cows are born with spaces in the gut that allow pathogens in. Without the colostrums the calf will not survive. Luckily the cow produces more than enough to allow it to be collected for human use.

Caprilic acid is also a natural antifungal, some people with gut issues may find this a little too irritating to be of use. This was my experience.

We also have used the master lemon cleanse to alkalinize our bodies. This will raise the ph and pathogens do not thrive in this environment. I have given directions elsewhere for the master lemon cleanse.

MORE ON LOW ADRENAL FUNCTION IN FM/CF SYNDROME

This is a quote from the Montague Hooper Report 1 May 2001:

"The endocrine system is uniquely disrupted in ME/CFS (52,53,54) A key feature is the demonstrated defect in HPA axis function (55.56) and patients are severely limited by the loss of dynamic hormone responses." "There is an abnormality of adrenal function and CT scans have shown that both the right and left adrenal glands are reduced by 50% when compared with controls.

The adrenals are responsible for many body functions. The most important may be that they provide the body with powerful stress hormone cortisol. Cortisol helps dial down pain levels, sharpens your mind, heightens mood, gives extra energy on demand, suppresses allergies and influences sleep cycle!

Again, No wonder people are suffering from fatigue, memory problems, sleep disturbance, need for daytime naps, weight gain especially belly fat! The adrenals are exhausted! The adrenals also stimulate the liver to produce glycogen which is stored over night and released to keep you from going into a low blood sugar and coma. The adrenals regulate blood pressure by secreting adrenaline! They also produce DHEA and testosterone which can be low in CF/FM.

Adrenals help fight fatigue, insomnia, infections, asthma, obesity and even thyroid problems. Too much cortisol is like searing acid which can eat away at delicate body tissues becoming toxic. You can also develop a metabolic weight loss syndrome when the adrenals are over producing adrenaline or cortisol. I once read that the reason people who get in severe sudden accidents actually die is from the rush of stress hormones to the gut; this actually is caused by the gut leaking into the whole body which becomes filed with sepsis. They then go into shock and coma. I found this interesting. Then is it any wonder that when we have a trauma or prolonged stress and continually have these same hormones going to the gut that this tissue becomes weak and hyper-permeable?

Long term stress can also run down the adrenal function and the adrenals become exhausted from wear and tear. Weight gain around the thighs or stomach can indicate the adrenals are sluggish!

The Wellness Resources has a couple products I think work well when you are under stress. The first one is "stress helper". This product contains (Pantethine, acetyl-l-carnitine, and carnosine) is provides energy producing cofactors to help the body cope with the demands of stress. They also help the body settle back into a more normal baseline of energy production once the stress is over, helping to avert wear and tear. Pantethine also improves mental clarity and supports adrenal function. Pantethine makes Coenzyme A (CoA) a pivotal nutrient in at least 70 energy-related metabolic pathways, including those that make adrenal hormones. You may take 300-1,800 mg of pantethine to help offset stress demands and support adrenal health.

Dr. Paul Cheney stated that you may detoxify these patients (CF/FM) but they may be left with defects in dynamic hypothalamus control, particularly of the dynamic hormones, cortisol and growth hormone. I was told by a physician who had CF/FM herself if you have low thyroid and adrenal function and it isn't addressed through intervention you can be left with permanent damage in the tissues. What Dr. Cheney says confirms this for me.

HEAVY METALS AND CF/FM

Metals can affect internal organs such as the thyroid and adrenals as well as liver and any tissue.

Magnesium deficiency is quite a common finding in conditions like fibromyalgia despite a high magnesium intake through the diet and supplementation. Muscle pain and spasms can occur as a result. Similarly, zinc deficiency due to malabsorption can result in hair loss or baldness as occurs in alopecia areata. Copper deficiency can occur in an identical way leading to high blood cholesterol levels and osteoarthritis, further bone problems develop as a result of the malabsorption of calcium, boron, silicon and manganese.

Metals can bind up enzymes which they are associated this prevents the cells from receiving the nutrition they need leading to nutrient deficiencies. Having high levels from over exposure of certain metals can also create nutritional imbalances within the body which might affect the health of connective tissues and joints.

Toxic metals may be sequestered deep in body tissues. They may only be revealed on a hair analysis after many months of nutritional therapy. It takes time to get the cells healthy enough to start to release them.

Fatigue is the prime symptom of a deficiency of adequate biochemical energy production in the body cells. Reduced energy production can be due to a wide range of factors including lack of rest, infection, chronic diseases, muscular tension, emotional upset and very often nutritional imbalances or deficiencies.

Magnesium is a catalyst for several hundred enzymes, including adenosine triphosphate or ATP. ATP is the molecule used as fuel for all cellular activity. Insulin production requires zinc and zinc and B-6 along with B-12 can be deficient in lead exposure.

One report I read stated that they felt FMS was a reflection of heavy metal contamination of the limbic system. When they used DMPS and procaine injections they clearly found elevated levels of urinary metal excretion.

This suggests that FMS is not only the limbic system but also the muscle and connective tissue is toxic.

A Scientific Report recently stated that metals and chemicals set off TNFa and Th1 type cytokine inflammatory responses as the T-cells and macrophages are activated. The cytokine response with Th1 and Th2 form the proof of cell damage and immune mechanism that poison the macrophage response. With time the Th1 process pulls the actual toxins into the lymph nodes when they bio-concentrate to the damaged node cells.

Mercury, nickel and uranium all cause a cytokine response via toxic metal damage to the cell. CHEMICALS ALSO CAUSE THE EFFECT, MAKING LYMPH NODE CELLS POISONED FROM MANY TOXINS SIMULTANEOUSLY!

Most important are metals and chemicals with long term internal retention in the body as these build up with time and cause long term effects in the lymph nodes. This sets off the nitric oxide and super-oxides activating cytokines inflammatory response.

I read a research paper that stated when lead comes up in the blood it can lead to M.S. I believe it causes many auto-immune conditions as well and have opinions stating that in deed this does happen! If you connect the dots this will ring true for you too!

HELPFUL TIPS FOR CF/FM

I was listening to Dr. Whitaker who is considered a leading authority on holistic or integrative medicine. I believe integrative medicine is the wave of the future. Doctors who are willing to learn about treatments that have been considered alternative in the past are helping their patients recover their health by side stepping side affects in many cases. I have read that even progressive hospitals are using alternative therapies to help their patients on the road to recovery.

Dr. Whitaker suggests that you use low dose naltrexone at night to help raise the endorphins which help us fight off pain.

He also suggested that you use L-carnitine which helps the cells produce energy within them and D-Ribose which is a natural sugar which can help boost energy in the cells.

Drinking pop is a real no no since phosphates can build up in the muscle tissue and contribute to pain. Caffeine is also an irritant to the gut so try to avoid tea and coffee until you get the gut healed. I was asked when first diagnosed if I drank diet soda. I didn't understand why I was asked this until recently when I read an article that said aspartame sensitizes the nerves to pain. I have also read that aspartame is a neurotoxin and a leading physician has testified before congress to this fact.

I recently read they are finding more violent outburst among teens who consume pop. I recently found a clue to this. Dr. David Brownstein recently wrote in his book, "Iodine Why You Need It Why You Can't Live Without It" that bromide toxicity has been reported from the ingestion of some carbonated drinks (e.g., Mountain Dew, AMP Energy Drink, some Gatorade products), which contain brominated vegetable oils. Bromide becomes toxic to the body by blocking receptors for iodine. This can affect the thyroid gland leading to fatigue and dysfunction.

The body's energy becomes blocked also from the toxicity in the mitochondria inside the cells that produce ATP. ATP is the body's energy source. When ATP is blocked, it interferes with energy, metabolism and heat in the body. Dr. Brownstein states, "if you treat with thyroid hormone without correcting for iodine deficiency, you will increase the body's need for iodine and worsen the iodine-deficient problem that is already present."

"When hypothyroidism is present, the body is in a hypometabolic state." "In other words, all bodily functions slow down and the consequences of this state include cold extremities, dry skin, fatigue, brain fog and weight gain." Fluoride and chlorine also block the iodine receptors. No wonder we have an epidemic of thyroid problems in this country.

For muscle pain, I use 2-3 tablespoons of ground ginger from my spice rack. Put it in 1-2 cups of water and boil until you can smell its essence then add it to your bath tub of water as hot as you can take it and soak until the water is cool. This helps release lactic acid that can build up in muscle tissues in an anaerobic metabolism state. I also use Epsom Salts to soak it has the same affect.

A warm lap blanket on cold winter nights helps a lot also!

FIBRIN LEVELS IN CF/FM

I found a research article that said there are high fibrin levels in both fibromyalgia and multiple sclerosis.

When I was first tested for this my fibrin levels were high, my doctor said it didn't mean anything but I have since learned that in Europe they had been looking at high fibrin levels as a marker for inflammation in the body for some time now. Doctors who have educated themselves are doing the same.

I have researched this and found this to be true; it does indicate a high level of inflammation. The body produces fibrin when it is trying to repair damage that is going on either by injury or free radical damage to the blood vessel linings. High fibrin levels can put you at higher risk for heart attack or stroke! I also learned that fibrin can build up in the small blood vessel linings and starve the underlying tissues for oxygen.

I have used Nattokinase to break down fibrin. It also helps lower fibromyalgia pain because it cleans up the small blood vessels.

C-reactive protein is also inflammatory; it is produced by the liver. The body creates inflammation to try and protect tissues from antigens (anything foreign to the body). They have found cytokines to be elevated in CF/FM.

Cytokines are also inflammatory. So yes there is a lot of inflammation going on sometimes but it isn't necessarily obvious to the eye.

Omega three fatty acids help counteract inflammation. I seem to do best with flax and evening primrose oil.

Of course healing a leaky gut also helps lower inflammation. Health Resources has a great product called "GI & Muscle Helper". It contains glutamine which is very healing. Glutamine is also a major component of muscle and is needed for muscle health. "GI & Muscle Helper" may be added to "Daily Protein" to boost muscle recovery from exercise.

N-Acetyl Glucosamine (NAG) is a key nutrient that helps form mucin within the digestive tract. Mucin is a muco-protein that acts as a lubricant, forming a natural barrier that helps protect the digestive lining. Adequate mucin supports healthy intestinal permeability, assisting digestion and absorption of food and nutrients.

You can also get L-glutamine in pill and powder form from the health food store. Two pills on empty stomach three times a day or one tsp.in water three times a day helps bring relief from leaky gut. I've also read taking this before going to bed is helpful!

LEAKY GUT SYNDROME

The well-validated IAG urine test is a test for an aberrant metabolite of tryptophan and if positive, is indicative of a malfunctioning and leaky gut; it indicates a compromised digestive process which in turn leads to opioid excess as a result of mal-digestion and uptake of opioid peptides derived from dietary sources. You may also ask for an Elisa Assay that measures the antibodies produced toward proteins.

The main culprits are well-known as being the opioid precursor peptides gluten and casein, with casein from cows milk causing more problems than casein from sheep's milk; they are broken down in the gut to opioid peptides, namely gliadomorphin and casomorphin and it is these which readily cross the damaged gut membrane and give rise to a cascade of multi-system problems. These "escaped" peptides are scientifically measurable in urinary peptide profiles.

Elaine Marie Graham

Significantly, if the gut is leaky, the same factors also cause the blood brain barrier to be leaky, with resultant effects of opioids on the central nervous system; this causes not only a local, but also a systemic reaction. Studies show this is not a genetic phenomenon but an acquired one. "There is now evidence from primary care of a surprisingly high frequency of unsuspected EMA test (endomysial antibodies) in people with non-specific symptoms." "We now suggest that screening for CD (celiac disease) be added to the short list of mandatory investigations in cases of suspected CFS". Both these factors may relate to the increased incidence of irritable bowel syndrome in ME/CFS, which is high: 73% as opposed to 22% of the general public.

Reference The Montague/Hooper Paper May 1, 2001 (Search Engine)

Without tryptophan, the body can't make serotonin which is necessary to stave off mood swings and depression.

Foods that deliver tryptophan are:

Eggs, cold water fish (salmon, tuna, anchovies, and mackerel) nuts, and seeds, soy, soy milk, tofu and soybeans, turkey and yogurt. These foods contain the amino acid tryptophan. Tryptophan also boosts levels of dopamine and norepinephrine. The supplement 5-http found in health food stores will deliver 5 hydroxyl tryptophan.

SUPPLEMENTS I HAVE FOUND HELPFUL IN FM/CF

Melatonin is something I have used to help me get to sleep on those nights I just knew it wasn't going to come easy. My experience was that when I took it a half hour before bed, I could easily go to sleep. I wasn't aware that it also has some benefit in synchronizing body rhythms but this would also be great for travelers because going from one time zone to another can really be hard on the bodies' natural clock.

I have used Wellness Resources Thyroid Helper. I have been on drugs to support my thyroid function since 2001. Sometimes even with drug supplementation the thyroid continues to be more and more sluggish. Since taking the Thyroid Helper product my thyroid function seems to have stabilized. My nurse practitioner seemed surprised by this but very elated.

Milk thistle supports liver function and dandelion is a tonic for weak digestion and gall bladder. R-Alpha Lipoic Acid has also shown to modulate NF-kappaB and is highly protective of liver function. Chlorella is high in anti-oxidant properties and a good detoxifier as is chlorophyll. Trans-Resveratrol supports anti-oxidant systems involved with detoxification, including the Phase II liver detox system and gastrointestinal glutathione peroxidase. N-Acetyl-Cycteine is central to producton of glutathione which has been found to be low in chronic fatigue syndrome. Taurine and Glycine support phase II detoxification and enchances bile flow. Taurine can be toxic to some people with certain genetic profiles, so be careful with this. Ornithine Alpha-Ketoglutarate helps maintain proper protein metabolism, supports clearance of ammonia. Ornathine is used in Phase II conjugation. We have used arginine and ornathine when doing a liver and gallbladder cleanse. Proteins from the leaky gut once in the blood can lead to gallbladder problems and gallstones. One of my favorite physicians, who was a young woman and very knowledgeable, said this was the reason I was developing gallstones.

Dr. Paul Cheney who has probably treated more people with chronic fatigue/fibromyalgia in the U.S.than any other physician stated that these people are loaded with chemicals, pesticides and heavy metals. He also suggested eliminating food intolerances and healing of the leaky gut. I'm sharing with you the products I have found to be most helpful for these problems. These include the above products along with colostrum and L-glutamine for healing the gut. Colostrum is a great aid for boosting a sluggish immune system. It can also modulate an over-active immune system. When my fibro pain would be in a flare up in the beginning of my illness, before I knew about L-glutamine, I used colostrum and I could immediately feel a difference in my pain level. I had a very over-active immune system due to the food intolerances along with no doubt the immune system reaction to antigens like metals. My husband and I both got a good benefit from the colostrum but it wasn't the total answer to our problems. Nor was it the answer for the friend that introduced us to it. I now believe the root of the problem is healing the mitochondria damage! Getting rid of toxins must come first!

I'm sure all anti-oxidants are helpful because there is a lot of free radical activity going on when you have chronic inflammation in the body. Quercetin is a great anti-oxidant and helps with congestion, helps with restful sleep, and modulates the behavior of the gene signal NF-kappa B. Quercetin is also an aid in optimal bone health. Mangosteen has helped with my chronic inflammation; it has a cox-II type inhibitor in it. You may not experience anything immediately but give it a little while and you will definitely feel the difference.

SYMPTOMS OF LEAD AND HEAVY METAL EXPOSURE DIAGNOSED AS CF/FM

I was stunned when I took a look at what the Centers for Disease Control charted as symptoms of lead poisoning. It took 7 years for a doctor to look at heavy metals in my case after being diagnosed with CF/FM and I had to seek out this doctor. It is a shame that doctors are missing these problems which contribute no doubt to bringing on CF/FM. Long term internal retention of metals causes a high degree of disability.

This comes under the title of "Health Effects to Lead Exposed Adults by Blood Lead Level" under the CDC's own websit:

If you have a level of:

5-9 pg/dl—Possible adverse population effects suggested by epidemiologic studies:

10-19 pg/dl—Possible spontaneous abortion, reduced newborn birth weight, possible blood pressure changes, and possible renal dysfunction.

20-39 pg/dl—Spontaneous abortion, reduced newborn birth weight, possible blood pressure changes, possible renal dysfunction, and possible non-specific symptoms. Headache, Fatigue, Sleep disturbances, constipation, diarrhea, arthralgia, myalgia, decreased libido, mood swings, personality changes, and possible CNS affects memory and attention deficits.

If any of these sound familiar or if you have been diagnosed with FM/CF you may want to have a chelation challenge to determine if you are dealing with heavy metals. Remember that it might require a number of months on nutritional therapy to mobilize some metals. I was on therapy for 8 months before things like bismuth started showing up in the hair analysis. I also had a nutritional evaluation and antimony showed up in the blood. No doubt my cells were mobilizing toxins. I had no doubt carried these metals for years but the major symptoms only showed up after I developed leaky gut and metabolic changes when I had an injury and lots of drugs.

After healing the gut and getting rid of the food intolerances, I started looking for other factors that were contributing to my problems and I found heavy metals at the heart of the matter. I was no doubt exposed to metals from the work I did.

When they looked at the umbilical cord blood levels of mothers who did lead soldering in Taipei they found all the metals associated with this soldering process. You can find information on this at Pub Med occupational exposure to lead or go to:

Wiley Online Library "Parental occupational lead exposure and lead concentration of newborn cord blood". The Material Safety Data Sheet from the manufacturer states "melted solder above 100 degrees farenheight will liberate toxic lead and or antimony fumes". Other routes of entry are skin, ingestion, inhalation and health effects are acute and chronic. No wonder I have suffered all these terrible symptoms and disability. Its only from doing my own research and taking control of my own health that I am here today. Many of you may need to take this route as well!

Metals can affect internal organs such as the thyroid and adrenals as well as liver and kidneys. Late effects can cause possible renal failure, encephalopathy of the brain, liver dysfunction and now they know it can throw off the methylation detox pathways that help the body convert homocysteine to methionine. Metals deplete nutrients because they bind the enzymes that deliver them to the cells. This leads to mal-nutrition. I have read that even one deficiency can lead to a disease process. I believe that God designed our foods to deliver all the nutrients we need when we eat a well balanced diet. He did not want us to die due to the toxic processes we are experiencing today. However industrial farming has stripped selenium, magnesium and iodine from our soils so many of our foods are lacking these nutrients.

My physician stated that we weren't meant to be exposed to all the metals we have been exposed to. He believes that the Industrial revolution has brought this problem about and I have to agree with his analysis of this problem.

Our genes are mutating due to the pressures of these extreme environment changes. I have no doubt that the explosion of autism is the result of the toxins that have been in our environment, foods, medicines and medical treatments. Like my very wise physician says "we weren't meant to deal with all the industrial chemicals that we are dealing with today." "Our genes can't keep up with the rapid changes in our environment."

Magnesium deficiency is quite a common finding in conditions like fibromyalgia despite a high magnesium intake through the diet and supplementation. Muscle pain and spasms can occur as a result. Similarly, zinc deficiency due to malabsorption can result in hair loss or baldness as occurs in alopecia areata. Copper deficiency can occur in an identical way leading to high blood cholesterol levels and osteoarthritis. Further, bone problems develop as a result of the malabsorption of calcium, boron, silicon and manganese.

Metals can bind up enzymes which they are associated with leading to nutrient deficiencies. The cells then become deficient in all kinds of trace minerals. I had a hair analysis in the beginning of my illness that showed not only a lack of certain nutrients but an imbalance in many nutrients. I had high copper levels so this can deplete zink. Imbalances in some nutrients can also cause problems in the muscles and joints.

Toxic metals may be sequestered deep in body tissues. They may only be revealed on a hair analysis after many months of nutritional therapy when the cells are able to mobilize them. I found this to be true. After about 8 months on nutritional therapy which included a liquid vitamin and mangostein. A hair analysis was repeated and the bismuth which was being released was showing in the hair analysis. The amount showing was off the chart which shows I was exposed to a lot of it. This is one of the elements in the soldering material. I don't know of any other source I could have encountered this problem. What I have learned is that when one element is really elevated other elements may not be showing. I felt really poorly when I was eliminating this element and I had really dark circles under my eyes. I thought about giving up on this whole process of trying to detox but I knew my health would only deteriorate if I didn't continue the process of trying to free myself from these toxins since my system is now very reactive to antigens. I feel the only choice is to continue to try and get rid of the antigens and improve my health. I also had a nutritional analysis that showed some antimony. This wasn't a challenge just a simple blood draw. This means I was releasing the antimony from the cells in to the blood.

Fatigue is the prime symptom of a deficiency of adequate biochemical energy production in the body cells. Reduced energy production can be due to a wide range of factors including lack of rest, infection, chronic diseases, muscular tension, emotional upset and very often nutritional imbalances or deficiencies; these can be caused by heavy metal exposures.

Magnesium is a catalyst for several hundred enzymes, including adenosine triphosphate or ATP. ATP is the molecule used as fuel for all cellular activity. Insulin production requires zinc and zinc and B-6 along with B-12 can be deficient in lead exposure.

One report I read stated that they felt FMS was a reflection of heavy metal contamination of the limbic system. When they used DMPS and procaine injections they clearly found elevated levels of urinary metal excretion.

This suggests that FMS is not only the limbic system but also the muscle and connective tissue is toxic.

Most important are metals and chemicals with long term internal retention in the body as these build up with time and cause long term effects in the lymph nodes. This sets of the nitric oxide and super oxides activating cytokines inflammatory response.

I read a research paper that stated when lead comes up in the blood it can lead to M.S. I have read it causes many auto-immune conditions as well and I have to believe this is true. If you connect the dots this will ring true for you too! All you have to do is look at the research.

HOLISTIC PHYSICIANS

I was listening to Dr. Witaker who is considered a leading authority on holistic or integrative medicine. I believe integrative medicine is the wave of the future. Doctors who are willing to learn about treatments that have been considered alternative in the past are helping their patients recover their health by side stepping side affects in many cases. I have read that even progressive hospitals are using alternative therapies to help their patients on the road to recovery.

Dr. Witaker suggests that you use low dose naltrexone at night to help raise the endorphins which help us fight off pain.

He also suggested that you use L-carnitine which helps the cells produce engergy within them and D-Ribose which is a natural sugar which can help boost energy in the cells. This however doesn't address low glutathione and mitochondria damage.

CAUSES OF LEAKY GUT SYNDROME

I want to share with you what the experts in the field are saying contribute to the development of this problem.

Dr. Zoltan P. Rona wrote back in 9/26/2009 that the follow contribute to the leaky gut: antibiotics because they lead to the overgrowth of abnormal flora in the gastrointestinal tract (bacteria, parasites, candida, fungi) Alcohol and caffeine (strong gut irritants)

Foods and beverages contaminated by bacteria like helicobacter pylori, klebsiella, citrobacter, pseudomonas and others.

Chemicals in fermented and processed food (dyes, preservatives, peroxidized fats)

Enzyme deficiencies (e.g. celiac disease, lactase deficiency causing lactose intolerance)

NSAIDS (non-steroidal anti-inflammatory drugs) like ASA, ibuprofen, indomethacin,

Prescription corticosteroids (e. g. prednisone)

High refined carboyhdrate diet (e.g. candy bars, cookies, cake, soft drinks, white bread)

Prescription hormones like the birth control pill mold and fungal mycotoxins in stored grains, fruit and refined carbohydrates.

There is new research that indicates an intolerance to gluten in grains may also cause "leaky gut."

The antibodies created by the leaky gut phenomenon against these antigens can get into various tissues and trigger an inflammatory reaction when the corresponding food is consumed or the microbe is encountered. auto-antibodies are thus created and inflammation becomes chronic. If this inflammation occurs in a joint, autoimmune arthritis (rheumatoid arthritis) develops. If it occurs in the brain, myalgic encephalomyelitis (a.k.a. chronic fatigue syndrome) may be the result. If it occurs in the blood vessels, vacuities (inflammation of the blood vessels) may be the result.

Dr. Scott Rigden wrote on 9/28/2009 article "Leaky Gut Syndrome and Fibromyalgia/Chronic Fatigue Syndrome": Articles in Lancet (341,491 1993) and the Annals of Allergy in 1990 summarize agents that commonly cause Leaky Gut Syndrome. These include bacterial infections, ethanol, food allergies, drugs, (antibiotics, NSAIDS and cortisone, xenobiotics, toxic heavy metals, stress, poor quality diet, parasites, yeast and viral infections.

Mercury may be one of the main offenders: There are ongoing discussions about the dangers of silver amalgam fillings in our teeth which are 50% mercury.

Other sources of mercury: vaccines, paints, broken thermometers and barometers, felt, fresh & salt water fish and shell fish, grains, seed treated with mercury fungicide, fabric softeners, adhesives, mercurial diuretics, ointments, antiseptics, floor waxes and polishes, wood preservatives, cinnabar, some cosmetics, film, photoengraving, tattooing, plastics, histology labs, industrial wastes, sewage sluge, sewage disposal, air and water in and around industrial areas, wiring devices/switch makers and manufacturers of measuring and control instruments.

In another chapter we will talk about chronic fatigue/ fibromyalgia and tests that you might want to have so keep reading. If you are dealing with this, it might save you a lot of pain and aggravation!!!!!!! ADDITIONAL INFORMATION ON LEAKY GUT SYNDROME

I would like to share with you an article I found by Dr. Gloria Gilbere. She stated, "I nearly died from the use of Naiads."

She states, "Our ancestors attributed maladies of unknown origins to evil spirits; today, we speak confidently about disease-generating microorganisms." "With modern invisible illness, an opinion not so different from that of our ancestors exists among some physicians, health practitioners, families, insurance companies, and employers who believe those suffering symptoms of multiple chemical sensitivity (MCS), fibromyalgia, some types of arthritis, chronic fatigue and myofascial pain syndromes must have some hidden demon that brings on these invisible disorders." "This is a classic case of blame the victim!"

"Fortunately, a different opinion is finally emerging—that disease is not a separate entity, but a changed state of the organism, an imbalance of natural equilibrium harmony of bodily systems that is caused by the accumulation of residues of toxic chemicals we are exposed in to in food, water, air consumer products, and environment." What is equally important to note is insight of the past decade declaring all diseases both genetic and environmental." Dr. Oz stated "our genes load the gun our environment pulls the trigger." I of course believe it is environment and blaming it on genes is an easy excuse for many things.

Much attention has been given to the small intestine in its connection to MCS, fibromyalgia and chronic fatigue syndrome, especially leaky gut syndrome (clinically known as intestinal permeability).

In leaky gut the villi of the small intestine are weakened and allow toxic material and food particles to permeate and enter the bloodstream. What is not often discussed is the leaking of toxic matter from the walls of the large intestine. The large intestine is intimately connected to the portal venous system of the liver through an elaborate network of large and small veins, and to the lymphatic system through the cisterna cilia. A more appropriate name for leaky gut should be auto-intoxication.

Due to pancreatic insufficiency, maintaining a cesspool of decaying toxic matter in the leaky gut (colon) is the process by which the body literally poisons itself. Many forms of "incurable" diseases get their start in the colon.

It is now believed that most pain and inflammation associated with MCS and inflammatory disorder occurs from build-up of toxins stored in the soft and connective tissue. Chronic use of NSAIDs, especially in high doses, increases the permeability of leaking of the colon according to Dr. Gilbere.

She recommends systemic oral enzymes to break up circulating immune complexes for reduction of pain and inflammation.

Natural pancreatic digestive enzymes are also helpful. Some may have an abnormal carbohydrate metabolism which can cause pyruvates in the blood. This is due to insufficient production of pancreatic digestive enzymes along with leaky gut syndrome.

Digestive enzymes help break down the food proteins etc. from the leaky gut that get in to the bloodstream.

I hope this information helps explain the mechanisms of the leaky gut syndrome and makes this topic a little clearer.

Dr. Scott Rigden wrote the "leaky gut is the cause of fibromyalgia and what causes this is drugs like naprosyn, cortisone, antibiotics, bacterias, parasites, and heavy metals."

When the leaky gut is present, high levels of small peptides cross the damaged gut membrane leading to changes in brain chemistry which have behavioral, cognitive, neurological, and endocrinological and immunological consequences This leads to opioid excess as a result of mal-digestion and uptake of opioids in the brain tissues.

Much attention has been given to the small intestine in its connection to MCS, fibromyalgia and chronic fatigue syndrome, especially leaky gut syndrome (clinically known as intestinal permeability).

In leaky gut the villi of the small intestine are weakened and allow toxic material and food particles to permeate and enter the bloodstream. What is not often discussed is the leaking of toxic matter from the walls of the large intestine. The large intestine is intimately connected to the portal venous system of the liver through an elaborate network of large and small veins, and to the lymphatic system through the cisterna cilia. A more appropriate name for leaky gut should be auto-intoxication.

Due to pancreatic insufficiency, maintaining a cesspool of decaying toxic matter in the leaky gut (colon) is the process by which the body literally poisons itself. Many forms of "incurable" diseases get their start in the colon.

It is now believed that most pain and inflammation associated with MCS and inflammatory disorder occurs from build-up of toxins stored in the soft and connective tissue. Chronic use of NSAIDs, especially in high doses, increases the permeability of leaking of the colon according to Dr. Gilbere.

She recommends systemic oral enzymes to break up circulating immune complexes for reduction of pain and inflammation.

Natural pancreatic digestive enzymes are also helpful. Some may have an abnormal carbohydrate metabolism which can cause pyrruvates in the blood. This is due to insufficient production of pancreatic digestive enzymes along with leaky gut syndrome.

Digestive enzymes help break down the food proteins etc. from the leaky gut that get in to the bloodstream.

I hope this information helps explain the mechanisms of the leaky gut syndrome and makes this topic a little clearer.

Dr. Scott Rigden wrote the "leaky gut is the cause of fibromyalgia and what causes this is drugs like naprosyn, cortisone, antibiotics, bacterias, parasites, and heavy metals."

When the leaky gut is present, high levels of small peptides cross the damaged gut membrane leading to changes in brain chemistry which have behavioral, cognitive, neurological, and endocrinological and immunological consequences This leads to opioid excess as a result of mal-digestion and uptake of opioids in the brain tissues.

Functional medicine physicians are now acknowledging that leaky gut syndrome is the root cause of fibromyalgia. Fibromyalgia was a name given to a group of symptoms most of which are centered in the muscles and nerves. Fibro refers to muscle tissue while myalgia is a name for muscle pain.

Dr. Zoltan P. Rona who is a medical doctor who went back to school to learn about alternative medicine spoke about the "leaky gut syndrome" back in the early 90's. Dr. Rona stated that "leaky gut syndrome is the name given to a very common health disorder in which the basic organic defect is an intestinal lining which is more permeable (porous) than normal". The abnormally large spaces present between the cells of the gut wall allow the entry of toxic material into the bloodstream that would, in healthier circumstances, be repelled and eliminated. The gut becomes leaky in the sense that bacteria, fungi, parasites and their toxins, undigested protein, fat and waste normally not absorbed into the bloodstream in the healthy state, pass through a damaged, hyper permeable, porous or "leaky" gut. This can be verified by special gut permeability urine tests, microscopic examination of the lining of the intestinal wall as well as the blood stream with phase contrast or dark field microscopy of living whole blood.

The "leaky gut" can lead to food intolerances which can be detected by an assay called the Elisa assay. This is a simple blood test that looks at how many antibodies might be produced for gluten, casein or any food protein. The leaky gut syndrome is almost always associated with autoimmune diseases such as fibromyalgia/chronic fatigue syndrome, lupus, alopecia areata, rheumatoid arthritis, polymyalgia rheumatica, multiple sclerosis, sjogrens syndrome, vitiligo, thyroiditis, vasculitis, crohn's disease, ulcerative colitis, urticaria (hives), diabetes and Raynaud's disease. Physicians are increasingly recognizing the importance of the gastrointestinal tract in the development of allergic or autoimmune disease according to Dr. Zoltan P. Rona.

The inflammation that causes the leaky gut syndrome also damages the protective coating of antibodies of the IgA family normally present in a healthy gut which are produced along the intestinal tract. Since IgA helps us ward off infections, with leaky gut problems we become less resistant to viruses, bacteria, parasites and candida.

Proteins that enter through the leaky gut can overwhelm the liver's ability to detoxify. This can result in symptoms such as confusion, memory loss, brain fog or facial swelling when the individual is exposed to a perfume or in cigarette smoke that he or she had no adverse reaction to prior to the development of the leaky gut syndrome.

Carrier proteins present in the gastrointestinal tract that are needed to transport minerals from the intestines to the blood are damaged by the inflammation process. For example, magnesium deficiency (low blood cell magnesium) is very common in fibromyalgia. Zink deficiency can occur in an identical way leading to high blood cholesterol levels and osteoarthritis. Bone problems develop as a result of malabsorption of calcium, boron, silicon and manganese. New research is indicating a much high mortality rate from all diseases when leaky gut is present.

Also in those with gluten intolerance the statistics have been quite startling for the increase in strokes and heart attacks.

MONTAGUE HOOPER PAPER MAY 2001

An enzyme designed to take out viruses becomes damaged and this shows up as low 37 kDa sized enzyme produced by calpain (an apoptotic enzyme) the whole process affects the calcium and potassium channel mechanism. A higher ratio of 37 kDa and 80 KDa enzymes is associated with more severe clinical symptoms in CFS.

Both abnormal RNaseL activity and low oxygen consumption were observed in most patients with CFS. Low tolerance for physical activity may be linked to poor oxygen transport by red blood cells due to free radical damage. The mitochondria of the cells also can become damaged by free radical activity. This prevents the process of converting proteins and sugars into energy within the cells.

Increased apoptosis (programmed cell death in peripheral blood monuclear cells has been suggested to contribute to the symptomology of CFS.

Baseline heart rate and plasma epinephrine were increased in CFS patients suggesting an activated sympatho-adrenal state. Sympathetic nervous system dysfunction is integral to CFS pathology.

Eighty five studies confirm autonomic nervous system dysfunction in 90% of CFS patients. This can result in changes of (blood pressure, pulse rate, breathing and body temperature). Substantial evidence that both the sympathetic and parasympathetic nervous system are abnormal in CFS.

When you experience visual changes, it is an indication that the connective tissue turnover time has been altered. This could be associated with low growth hormone and low collagen production.

There is evidence of a degenerative process of muscle tissue in CFS as occurs in myopathies. This may contribute to muscle fatigability and it supports an organic origin for CFS.

One virus which is known to activate the coagulation system is the HHV-6. I'm sure others may be capable of triggering the same response as the immune system becomes activated.

Environmental influences which researchers worldwide are investigating include the frequent pairing of CFS with food and chemical sensitivities.

The RNaseL pathway is a series of enzymatic reactions which go on inside white blood cells when they perceive themselves to be challenged by viruses and possibly also by some toxic exposures.

SIMILARITIES FOUND IN AUTISM AND CHRONIC FATIGUE SYNDROME

After learning about a similarity between autism and chronic fatigue, I felt this information needs to go out to everyone.

I have been researching for information on blocks in the methylation systems since I have had difficulty in riding my system of heavy metals.

I found a research article that really explains so much about how the body detoxes. If you put "Suggestions for Treatment of Chronic Fatigue Syndrome based on the Glutathione Depletion—Methylation Cycle Block

Hypothesis for the Pathogenesis of CFS" by Richard A Van Konyenburg, Ph.D. in your search engine you will find this information.

They have found that glutathione is depleted in autism as it is in chronic fatigue syndrome. This is important because glutathione is an anti-oxidant produced by the body to help the body rid itself of toxins.

My glutathione levels have been very low when they tested me. I recently had a test by Nutrigenomics which looks at blocks in the methylation system. This is expensive and not covered by insurance but I felt it necessary to identify where I'm having problems in the detox pathways. I know I have had an imbalance in the liver detox pathways after having a caffeine liver challenge which identified this. Metals can damage the P450 enzyme that helps the liver detox! The clinical explanation said that this imbalance in the liver comes from drugs and metal exposures. I found this out several years after the test was done when I asked for the clinical explanation.

They give you high doses of caffeine and then look at the urine to see how fast the liver is detoxing it. I got a severe headache with this so I knew I wasn't detoxing well. There are several processes involved with methylating toxins. My physician says the first cycle of methylating is always off in people with fibromyalgia. All three of my processes were off after I had a IV challenge that didn't go well. I believe this was due to the fact I was low on several nutrients. My physician says he has had other patients that came from other doctors that have had this problem. He says he now checks everyone's nutritional status and ability to methylate toxins before trying any detox IV. Many M.D.s do not use this test but they should; it is very diagnostic and can pinpoint where the detox pathway may be off. Metals are also nortorious for blocking enzymes that carry nutrients so it isn't surprising that someone who has had these problems for a while will be nutritionally deficient.

Food intolerances go along with fibromyalgia because of the leaky gut. They have also found children with autism have intolerances to gluten and dairy in many instances. Healing of the gut is necessary to reverse food intolerances and L-glutamine is the best thing I have found for this. I was told to take 2 pills on an empty stomach three times a day in between meals. I also use the powder which has no taste in water or juice. I read in a book written by a physician that he also uses L-glutamine to help heal the children with autism!!!!!

When I was at my worst period with the food intolerances, I felt like this must be what it is like to be autistic, because the brain fog was so severe I could hardly function. Processing thoughts and memory were very impaired. I therefore believe this information could really help those who are dealing with autism, and possibly even ADHD.

I wrote researches of autism and asked them to investigate the link between autism and food intolerances after learning that one mother turned her son around in short order with colostrum and a change of diet which included taking gluten and dairy off the menu. It is now known that they are in deed dealing with digestive problems and food intolerances.

I found a great book called "Mastering Leptin" by Byron J. Richards, CCN with Mary Guignon Richards. I had never heard of the master hormone leptin and had no clue what it did or how it was made in the body. These authors are great!

MUSCLE CELL DAMAGE IN CF/FM

Byron J. Richards, CCN with Mary Guignon Richards have a book that is called "Mastering Leptin" "Your Guide to Permanent Weight Loss and Optimum Health". They have a chapter in the book on fibromyalgia. I haven't found anyone who understands the cause of the muscle pain like they do!

On page 236, they mention that high levels of location end product modified proteins (AGE) are created. This induces tissue damage once the antioxidant reserves of the muscle are used up. They say, "the proteins of the muscle fibers become cemented together in abnormal structures and no longer work properly." "This damage activates excess production of NF-kappaB which contributes to the pain and perpetuates the damage." "When nerve pain is initially directed at the muscles, the muscles activate their cellular defense mechanisms in an effort to withstand the problem." "As the problem continues, the antioxidant defense system is used up." "At this point, excess NF-kappaB is activated in an inflammatory manner. This in turn causes a progression of the local tissue damage and resulting pain."

The longer a person stays in FM pain, the more likely it is that damage is done to the muscles.

In low leptin states, the body is in a stressful wasting condition. There is excess cortisol fueling the wasting away of the body. This state of physical breakdown involves the excess production of TNFa and IL-6.

However, this time . . . these highly inflammatory immune signals do not come from the excess fat, they come from the cortisol and/or disease fueled wasting process. To reverse the effects of this process it is suggested in the book to take 2grams-6 grams of fish oil which will stop the wasting syndrome. It is also helpful to take evening primrose oil along with the fish oil. You can also substitute flax oil for the fish oil if you are concerned about their purity. Zinc is also important in anorexic metabolism wasting. Zinc can be depleted as well as B-6 from lead exposure and probably many other metals!

IMPORTANCE OF DIGESTIVE SYSTEM PROBLEMS IN CF/FM

Stress, alcohol, drugs, sugar and other refined foods over stimulate the pancreas and impair its ability to carry out important functions of making digestive enzymes. If the pancreas does not neutralize the acid coming from the stomach with bicarbonates, the proteolytic enzymes are destroyed. This can result in incomplete or "foreign" protein molecules being absorbed into the bloodstream and circulating throughout the body. These proteins are notorious for causing all types of allergic reactions, in particular those related to breathing and skin irritation.

Digestion of food in the stomach takes place at a ph of about l.8 to 3 (very acidic). When food enters the small intestine, the digestive process continues, but the area changes to an alkaline environment with a PH ranging from around 6.8 to as high as 9.

At the point where the acidic food leaves the stomach and enters the small intestines, the pancreas dumps in an alkalizing bicarbonate solution to neutralize the stomach's acid.

The pancreas also produces and secretes proteolytic enzymes that break down proteins into smaller components called amino acids. From these amino acids your body creates other enzymes, hormones and body tissue for growth and repair. Proteolytic enzymes also help regulate and control inflammation.

L-glutamine which is a simple amino acid can be found at the health food store. It has shown to be a great supplement for healing the mucosal lining and alleviating inflammation. I use it to help with any digestive upset. I shared this with my step-sister who had been struggling for months with digestive problems and was on a lot of medications for it. She is now off her meds and is feeling much better. They couldn't even find the ulcers when she went back for a check up.

METABOLIC ORIGIN OF CHRONIC FATIGUE/FIBROMYALGIA

Biopsies conducted on FMS patients indicate damage in mitochondria in the muscle, a metabolic abnormality. An impairment in glycolysis leads to an "energy crisis" with abnormal carbohydrate metabolism and phosphorylation, causing failure of thiamine activation and serotonin depletion.

Blood chemistry findings in FMS patients typically show:

Low:
Thiamine activation
Serotonin
Growth Hormone
High-Energy Phosphates (ATP) in Red Blood Cells

Lactic Dehydrogenase
Phospocreatinine-inorganic Phosphates
Phosphate/Creatinine/ATP
Magnesium
Tryptophan (plasma)
Cortisol
DHEAS
NADP (RBC)
Serum Serotonin, Norephinephrine and Dopamine (in cerebrospinal fluid)

High:
Pyruvates—this indicates abnormal carbohydrate metabolism. You may need more digestive enzymes to break down these carbs which is amylase, this also may be related to leaky gut syndrome.

Pyruvate/Lactase
Quinolinic Acid
Substance P—elevated in spinal cord which is a chemical messenger for pain signals to the brain and increases sensitivity to pain

Dr. Bellanti's study indicated that 75 percent of CFS subjects showed elevated levels of a major breakdown metabolite product of serotonin.

It has been estimated that 14 million people between the ages of 17-69 are affected by chronic fatigue syndrome. George Birkmayer M.D.Ph.D. first discovered the therapeutic application of NADH in cellular development and energy transmission. NADH is a naturally occurring coenzyme that activates bodily energy production. Results of an FDA approved, double-blind, placebo-controlled cross-over study published in February 1999 issue of Annals of Allergy, Asthma and Immunology found that CFS patients taking ENADA, a dietary supplement, were four times more likely to show improvements compared to those taking a placebo.

It has been found that growth hormone secretion regulated the rate of collagen production and this hormone has been found by Oregon researcher Robert Bennett M.D. to be on the low side in most people with FMS.

It isn't hard to see that nutrient deficiencies could be at the heart of a wide range of metabolic problems associated with chronic fatigue/fibromyalgia but only integrative or holistic doctors are trained to look for these problems. Could it be that even more diseases and disorders are brought about by nutrient deficiencies?

I can tell you first hand that the anxiety, depression and pain caused by pyrroles in the blood can be debilitating. This can be caused by lead exposure and stress. Many people had high lead levels before lead was removed from gasoline!!!!!!!!! Most people have never heard of this!!!!!! I have read that blood lead levels were in the mid teens before they took the lead out of gasoline in the early 80s. This was confirmed by Dr. Gary Gordon a leading authority on chelation therapy in a recent video he made on U-tube. People's blood lead levels have gone down substantially since the removal of lead from gasoline. They say it went down to 1-2 pg/dl. Since the bones and tissues are already toxic for these exposures, it doesn't take a lot of occupational exposure to cause lead poisoning. Lead can be stored in bone and soft tissues for up to 30 years and may be released back into the blood stream under times of stress or calcium deficiency.

HEAVY METALS AND CF/FM

If you visit the Center for Disease Control website you will find that they relate chronic fatigue to an endpoint of a disease resulting from multiple precipitating causes. Conditions that have been proposed to trigger the development of CFS include virus infection or other transient traumatic conditions, stress, and toxins.

The Agency for Toxic Disease Registry says "the over-toxicity causes extensive free radical damage"; inhibits cellular function, disrupts energy production by the mitochondria. Consequently the primary energy the cells produce is anaerobic which leads to extensive lactic acid buildup in the cells and more toxicity. Free radicals also cause oxidative stress to the mitochondria which is responsible for making energy within the cells.

The hypothalamus is injured and causes problems with every hormone in the body. This leads to metabolic disorders which doctors have failed to recognize in the past.

It is known that heavy metals inhibit the cytochrome P450 enzymes and mitochondrial energy production and that they are neuro-toxins. They also cause an acidic environment in the body which encourages the growth of bacterias and viruses. You can find PH strips from the pharmacy to check your PH levels in the urine and saliva. You may have to ask the pharmacist for these, they come with instructions.

Many nutrients can be displaced by metals. Zinc is displaced by cadmium, nickel, lead and mercury. B-6 and zink are displaced by lead. Lead can also interfere with the production of red blood cells. This can lead to pyrroles being excreted in the urine. This can be diagnosed through a urine test. This condition can be physically debilitating and cause severe anxiety, mood swings, depression and other neurological disorders. It also causes pain in the extremities such as the hands and feet, muscle and joint pain.

Nickel has been related to failure to thrive, mortality in animal studies, Lupus and chronic fatigue.

We mentioned earlier about burning of coal by electric power plants causes tons of mercury, arsenic, lead and cadmium are released into the atmosphere. This can contaminate food sources, water and air. Many people who work in an industrial setting are also routinely exposed to metals.

Power plants create two-thirds of the nation's sulfur dioxide emissions, which cause the acid rain that kills trees and pollutes lakes. They also produce a quarter of the nitrogen oxides that make smog; about 35 percent of mercury, which contaminates fish and can cause brain damage in fetuses if eaten by pregnant women, and about 40 percent of carbon dioxide, which contributes to global warming according to the Environmental Protection Agency.

SUGGESTED TESTS FOR CF/FM

Since it has been indicated that bacteria and viruses can attack the gut leading to "leaky gut syndrome", it would be wise to have a comprehensive digestive stool analysis. The stool analysis grows out all the bacteria, yeast and fungus etc. that might be in the stool culture and allows the pathologist to diagnose what might be contributing to irritation of the gut lining. Keep in mind that toxins can lower the immune system resistance to many pathogens. Metals may encourage yeast and bacterias etc.

There are new diagnostic test which have come from Europe that are identifying antibodies along the mucosal linings that may contribute to "leaky gut snydrome". Insurances aren't presently covering the cost but it may be well worth it to find out if your digestive complaints are related to intolerance to gluten. Gluten is the fibrous part of the grain which is 10 times higher than it was 100 years ago due to genetically modified grains.

In people with non-celiac gluten intolerance, the immune system attacks the gluten. It's basically a case of mistaken identity. The immune system sees gluten as a bacteria or virus and mounts a full-scale war. To do so, it produces an arsenal of antibodies to launch against whatever gluten you've ingested—even if it's a tiny amount. Every time gluten is eaten by someone with intolerance to it, the immune system whips itself into a frenzy. Over time, gluten-induced inflammation seeps throughout the body, this can lead to chronic disease. It has been said that a substance called zonulin is produced that pries apart the cells of the intestinal lining allowing bits of undigested food to scoot into the bloodstream, thus "leaky gut" is developed.

The immune system reacts to undigested food as if it were a bacteria or virus; it reacts by producing cytokines (produced by the immune system) which flood the body causing a ripple of inflammation.

In 2002 a New England Journal of Medicine review linked 55 different disorders to eating gluten, including anemia, epilepsy, type l diabetes and cystic fibrosis. This is confusing to doctors and they may be treating symptoms of gluten intolerance without knowing it.

One of the most sensitive tests to these antibodies is the tissue transglutaminase. If you've got them, chances are you've also got celiac. If tests are negative, but you still have symptoms you may want to get a genetic test which is a swab inside of the cheek to determine if you have a genetic predisposition for celiac disease.

You may also have an Elisa assay that looks for IgG and IgA antibodies to gliadin. It is a sign but not a certain indication that the body is in some way hostile to gluten. If you have leaky gut you may react to gliadin and casein most strongly but have other intolerances as well.

A 2009 study in the Journal of the American Medical Association found an increase risk of death among patients with both celiac and other types of gluten-related inflammation. The risk of mortality, mostly from heart disease and cancer (two leading inflammatory conditions), was an alarming 39 percent higher in people with celiac disease and a jaw-dropping 72 percent higher in people with gluten-related inflammation.

It has been estimated that 30 percent of northern Europeans (those who lived farthest from the origination of dietary grains in Mesopotamia) carry the genes for gluten intolerance.

Leaky gut syndrome can also allow mycoplasmas to enter the blood stream and there are laboratories that tests for these microbes.

The Fibromyalgia Network newsletter had an article in July 1997 that identified an enzyme found in joint diseases also elevated in fibromyalgia. This is the NTPPhase enzyme and may reflect the amount of joint destruction occurring in a person with this disorder as the tendons and ligament tissues are affected.

As the immune system is weakened by chemicals and toxic exposures, viruses can gain a foothold and contribute to fatigue and pain. Viruses that have been associated with CFS/ME and FMS are Human Herpes Virus-6 Cytomeglovirus and Epstein Barr Virus, and of course HIV has its own set of problems.

Problems to the mitochondria of the cells have been identified due to damage from oxidative stress or free radical damage. There are ongoing studies with a product called NT Factor which helps to heal the mitochondria. When the mitochondria are damaged the cells cannot properly produce energy and this leads to severe fatigue in CF/FM.

FOOD INTOLERANCES AND CHRONIC FATIGUE/FIBROMYALGIA

Many people have intolerances to foods of which they are not aware. It has been estimated that 60% of all undiagnosed miseries involve some form of food intolerance. Statistically you would be unusual if you didn't have one. It may be a food you never expected. It can be brought on by "leaky gut" syndrome". See articles on leaky gut.

Many people are becoming intolerant to gluten (grains, barley, oats and rye)

Here are a few of the common symptoms:

Arthritis, Asthma, Duodenal ulcer, Weight gain, Incontinence, Eczema, Bladder infection, lower back pain, Edema, Headaches, Diabetes types 1 & 2 they believe gluten intolerance may contribute to this as well as the GAD's antibody to dairy, Bronchitis, Depression, Bursitis, Diarrhea, Fatigue, Hyperactivity, Hypoglycemia, Learning Disability, Sinus Trouble, Irritable colon, Lupus, Multiple sclerosis, Recurrent infections.

What can you do for this? See the article on "Leaky Gut Syndrome" in one of my earlier articles. Wellness Resources has a good GI helper that contains L-glutamine. L-glutamine is a natural amino acid (protein) which many physicians are now recommending as a therapy to heal the leaky gut. I use it any time my stomach feels upset and it calms it right down. Go to http://www.chronicfatiguefibromyalgiawrongdiagnosis.com Wellness Resources upper right hand corner of page.

Once you develop gluten intolerance you may have to avoid it for life. If you don't, you can cause damage to the villi in the intestinal lining that absorb your nutrients. Thus you may become nutrient deficient and literally be starving even though you are eating a sufficient diet.

To avoid gluten you may have to visit a health food store to find gluten free breads and goodies. Some bakeries are now making it available and I believe this trend will continue as more people become aware of the problem and seek out gluten free products.

A new test has been developed to identify people who might develop celiac. Higher levels of Glo-3A found to be present is thought to be a bio-marker of impaired immune tolerance and increased gut permeability! TTG is an enzyme which alters gliaden molecule by changing glutamine residues, these bind to antigen presenting cells and activate T cells. This leads to damage to the villi that pull out nutrients from our digested food. This leads to malabsorption, gastrointestinal bloating and diarrhea. By the time TTG antibodies are detected, villous atrophy has already begun. We need to push to have these life saving tests covered by insurance companies and medicare. I was denied testing because they said the tests were too expensive and the treatment is the same—avoid gluten but I would really like to know if healing the gut resolved the problem!

My holistic physician suggested I use blueberry concentrate which will help to rebuild the villi. This does help with absorption and assimilation. I would recommend it to everyone.

Cherries and raspberries also have anothocyanadins which have been said to deliver more anti-inflammatory relief than aspirin. Maybe this is why they recommend cherry juice concentrate to people with arthritis. Olive oil acts like an anti-inflammatory. Ginger is also known to help tighten the spaces between the villi that might allow pathogens in to the system. Ginger is also a great anti-inflammatory. It has been recommended for people with joint pain to take ginger pills every day. I think juicing some carrots, golden apples and ginger is a great anti-inflammatory.

One researcher, Jonathan Forester M.D. said increases in levels of polyunsaturated fatty acids had the highest correlation with both fatigue and muscle pain scores. There has been a move by government to lower the polyunsaturated fats in processed foods but a lot of them probably still contain polyunsaturated fats. You'll want to be sure and check the potato chips. I have practiced good eating habits for years.

One reason for CFS patient's intolerance of sugar is the coexistence of yeast or bacterial overgrowth in the intestines. Foods most likely to cause a chemical reaction within the body are wheat, yeast, milk, sugar, peanuts, corn, eggs, citrus fruits, soy products, caffeine, alcohol, food additives preservatives and flavorings.

Foods usually well tolerated are nutritious poultry, fish, most fruits, vegetables, brown rice and plain yogurt with active cultures. Omega fats are recommended I prefer flax and evening primrose because of risk of contamination.

NECK INJURY AND FIBROMYALGIA

There have been lawsuits over neck injuries that lead to fibromyalgia, but the judicial system decided there were too many factors that can lead to the development of this condition so they stopped allowing these cases to go forward in workers comp cases.

I think the literature would indicate that injury to the neck can bring on damage to nerves of the spine. If any nerve becomes inflamed it can send pain along to other nerves which could involve the whole nervous system once this is initiated. My chiropractor said that if the skull is rotated and the nerves are stressed it can cause symptoms all the way down the spine. I'm sure this is true as I have experienced this myself after developing the neck strain.

Dr. Robert Gerwin M.D. described a phenomenon in which local muscle cell injury can stimulate the trigeminal nerve that leads to and from the brain. This stimulation of the trigeminal nerve may cause the neurons that travel to other muscle groups to become more sensitized to touch; thus, referring the pain elsewhere. As this situation ensues, a person may be more susceptible to developing painful trigger points in areas unrelated to the original site of the muscle injury.

Dr. Frank Porreca of the University of Arizona in Tucson, said "70% of your opioid receptors are located in the periphery (organs, muscles and other tissues) or at the level of the spinal cord juncture before the dorsal horn." "Only 30 % are located in the dorsal horn and brain."

"This is important to keep in mind, because under acute pain situations, opiates like morphine and codeine will work on those opioid receptors in the periphery to reduce the pain."

According to Ron Dubner, Ph.D. of the University of Maryland in Baltimore, "pain that persists for every day leads to changes in the central nervous system." "The changes result in amplification and increased sensation of pain."

This should be enough to get someone with a work related injury a substantial compensation, but don't count on it. President George Bush changed the laws governing worker's comp to exclude strain injuries. There seems to have been a steady assault on worker's rights over the last 20 years.

Jonathan Forester M.C. wrote in his book "Conquering CF, "In one study FM developed in over 20% of patients who had neck injuries." "Pain may result from a ruptured disc, spinal stenosis (narrowing in the spinal canal) thoracic outlet syndrome (narrowing where the nerves exist from the first rib) neuropathy or neuritis (a sick nerve)."

He also wrote, "Researchers found proinflammatory cytokines elevated as much as 4 fold." "Substance P, nerve growth factor and tumor necrosis factor-alpha appear to be vital in the pathophysiology of this illness." "Neurotransmitters such as norepinephrine and serotonin are low in the spinal fluid thus implicating these substances in the process as well." "Inflammatory cytokines are not elevated in depression or anxiety."

They now refer to worker's rights and human rights as "entitlements" as if to say that they aren't entitled to compensation, yet congress votes themselves in permanent salaries even after they leave office and permanent health care, now that is an entitlement!!! It seems we have become what Thomas Jefferson called an oligarchy. We are ruled by the few who slant the laws in their favor and do not consider the rights of the working people. I think it is time for a wake up call!!!! I recently read that senator's children do not have to pay back college tuition. Now that is an entitlement!!!!!!!!!! It should be eye opening when you think you are expected to work until 65 and they want to raise it even higher and they serve one term and have lifetime salary and benefits, including health care. They never have to worry about becoming disabled or out of money ever again. They never have to fight for long term disability, worker's comp or social security benefits.

They seem to favor laws that benefit disability insurance companies more than the people who have paid in to these programs. President Obama said he was going to try and correct the fact that for two decades people who have become disabled haven't been able to get their benefits. My insurrer was ordered to open hundreds of claims they closed that were questionable. I was told they sent out a letter in 2006 to claimants. I was on the reconsideration list but because I didn't receive this letter and didn't respond they closed my file and refused to reopen it! When I spoke to one of their employees they said a lot of people were saying they hadn't gotten that letter. I wonder how many actually did receive it and how many may have heard "you didn't reply so we closed your file". There were no laws governing disability for fibromyalgia when I became disabled, but there were laws governing chronic fatigue syndrome which were ignored by the company and insurance carrier. I didn't know back then that I had been exposed to the heavy metals.

RESEARCH PAPERS CONCERNING DISABILITY

While doing my research over the past sixteen years, I have been privileged to come across several very helpful articles especially if you're fighting for disability. It occurred to me that some of you might benefit from this information.

The first is a copy of a House of Representatives bill regarding fibromyalgia that was done in June of 1999. This bill recognizes the severity of this problem and some of the contributing factors which are stress, trauma, or possibly an infectious agent in susceptible people. Let us not forget that the top treating physician in the U.S., Dr. Paul Cheney said these people are loaded with all kinds of chemicals, pesticides and heavy metals and have to be detoxed before they will see improvement. I have a copy of his report.

The Fibromyalgia Network put out a report dated Jan. '92 that stated. "Four studies have said that fibromyalgia syndrome (FMS) can be as disabling as rheumatoid arthritis (RA). "One would think that based on these three studies alone, the disability issue on FMS was an open and closed case." "FMS subjects also experienced the same level of problems as RA individuals in areas of mobility, walking and bending, arm function, household tasks, social activities, exercise, fatigue, work, mood and health perceptions."

The Fibromyalgia Syndrome Political Case Statement Fibromyalgia Network l/96 states, "Researchers have noted a significant overlap between FMS and Chronic Fatigue syndrome (CFS) and a majority of patients who meet the diagnostic criteria for FMS also meet the CDC criteria for CFS."

I suggest you sign up for the Fibromyalgia newsletter with the Fibromyalgia Network; it has been helpful in finding some answers.

IMPAIRMENTS IN CHRONIC FATIGUE/FIBROMYALGIA

Are you trying to get disability? You need to know what the guidelines are for qualifying for disability.

Here are the medically determinable Impairments required to qualify for CFS and FMS.

One or more of the following must be documented for at least six consecutive months:

a. Palpably swollen or tender lymph nodes on exam
b. Nonexudative pharyngitis (sore throat without sings of inflammation)
c. Persisting, reproducible muscle tenderness on repeated examinations, including the presence of positive tender points
d. There is considerable overlap of symptoms between CFS and FMS, but individuals with CFS who have tender points have a medically determinable impairment. Individuals with impairments that fulfill the ACR criteria for FMS which includes the minimum number of tender points) may also fulfill the criteria for CFS. HOWEVER, individuals with CFS who do not have the specified number of tender points to establish FMS may still be found to have a medically determinable impairment.

The following tests may be used to help establish a medically determinable impairment in individuals with CFS (and FMS if they meet the criteria):

a. Elevated antibody to EBV capsid antigen equal to or greater than l:5120, or early antigen equal to or greater than l:640
b. An abnormal MRI scan of the brain
c. Neurally mediated hypotension as shown by tilt table testing or another clinically acceptable for of testing
d. Other tests, such as abnormal sleep studies or exercise intolerance

There are 18 specific tender points which will be noted in FM but you don't need all of them to have FM. Also check out the information under tests you should have.

Please ask for all tests results and keep a file for them where you can easily access them if you need to go for a hearing.

Check out the Disability Digest for more help in obtaining disability. It is free to become a member.

The following was found in the Montague/Hopper Paper from 2001:

Both baseline heart rate and plasma epinephrine were increased in CFS patients, suggesting an activated sympathy-adrenal state. Sympathetic nervous system dysfunction is integral to CFS pathology.

Both the sympathetic and parasympathetic nervous systems are abnormal in CFS.

I suggest this happens when you are exposed to chemical and metal toxins!

ARE YOU DISABLED BY CHRONIC FATIGUE/FIBROMYALGIA

Have you been disabled by chronic fatigue/fibromyalgia? If so you'll want to visit the Disability Digest forum.

Here you can learn about Lupus or Fibromyalgia and join the Disability Digest to learn about your disability. You can also find legal help on how to obtain social security income. Learn about housing for the disabled. And if you need to try and make a little additional income they can advise you on the best path to take to achieve this.

Membership is free and you can also become an affiliate for free!

You can have test to look at genetic profile and detox systems at Genova Diagnostics Lab at http://www.gdx.net. She also has tests that look at the methylation system to see if there needs to be support there.

She has come up with protocols for chronic fatigue/ fibromyalgia as well as autism. You can also go to Dr. Gary Gordon's website he has a program to help people dealing with mercury and other toxic exposures. He calls this his F.I.G.H.T. program.

He said in his video he was ill from mercury exposure until he was 29. He also had problems with the methylation system. He has first hand experience with the disabling side of this exposure. He has come up with a step program that includes getting rid of infections, addressing hormone imbalances, addressing food intolerances, healing the gut and getting rid of heavy metals and other toxins. He has products that he has available which he uses in his practice. You might also find him by looking up the "lyme" doctor.

I have come across some really great sites that research the connection of heavy metal exposure and CF/FM. If they don't come up by using the address then do a search and you should find them by topic.

I decided to share the URL for these sites here:

Fibromyalgia Syndrome and Heavy Metal Toxicity by Dietrich Klinghardt, MD, Ph.D. There are actual case studies of metal toxicity and the development of FM here!

ATSDR Agency for Toxic Substances and Disease Registry
http://www.atsdr.cdc.gov/substances/ToxOrganSystems.asp

Multiple Sclerosis
http://imva.info/index.php/mercury-medicine/multiple-sclerosis/

The Weight of Lead: Effects Add Up in Adults
http://elcosh.org/en/document/990/d000945/the-weight-of-lead%253A-effects-add-up-in-adults.html

CF/FM syndrome, Scleroderma, Lupus, MCS: the mercury connection. B. Windham
http://www.flcv.com/cfsfm.html

Eleven pages of eye opening research on metals and disease!

Remember Dr. Cheney who has treated over 3,000 CF/FM patients says you have to detox these people of toxins and heavy metals and get rid of the food sensitivities to see results!!!!!!! You can search Dr. Zoltan P. Rona's site also he said it is leaky gut that is at the heart of FM/CF. He says also that if the thyroid and adrenal are out for some time you might lose control over the adrenals. He has a lot of information on many health disorders at his site!

You may be wondering why your energy levels just won't stay up or even crash.

The fatigue of a 45 year old woman with FMS is approximately twice the fatigue of a 67 year old patient with rheumatoid arthritis. This symptom could lead to a diagnosis of chronic fatigue.

What could be causing these very frustrating and sometimes scary episodes of not being able to function?

Have you ever heard of the Krebs energy cycle? You might want to do some research on this subject. I won't bore you with all the technical aspects of this, but just tell you that basically it has to do with how your cells take in nutrients and glucose and convert it to energy. In fibromyalgia/chronic fatigue the mitochondria of the cell can be damaged. These are the little power houses that convert nutrition to energy. When these mitochondria are not working you can feel the full force of chronic fatigue.

There are supplements out that are trying to address the healing of the mitochondria but if you still have an acid PH or are not able to get rid of chemicals and metals you may have trouble seeing progress.

Stirring up toxins while trying to detox may create some further damage to the cells through free radical damage. I have read suggestions that you take extra anti-oxidants while trying to detox. I have done this myself and my recent Bio 101 test showed good results. I am still however dealing with damage to the mitochondria.

SCIENTIFIC INFORMATION ON METALS

They state: (heavy metals and chemicals) set off TNFa and Th1 Type cytokine inflammatory responses as the T-cells and macrophages are activated. The cytokine response with Th1 and Th2 form the proof of cell damage and immune mechanism that poison the macrophage response. With time the Th1 process pulls the actual toxins into the lymph nodes, when they bio-concentrate to the damaged node cells.

Many toxic metals set off the cell toxic response and metals like mercury, nickel, and uranium all cause a cytokine response via toxic metal damage to the cell. Chemicals also cause the effect, making lymph node cells poisoned from many toxins simultaneously.

Most important are metals and chemicals with long term internal retention in the body as these build up with time and cause long term effects in the nodes, setting of continual nitric oxide and super oxides and activating the cytokines inflammatory response. Thus causing long term problems like insoluble oxides in the lungs and lymph nodes. The continual activation of the cytokines in the body cause cell damage effects in all tissues.

The Th1 activation often begins with asthma, rashes, and allergy symptoms as indicators.

With the acid PH this creates in the body the cells become leaky which deposits calcium in muscle tissue!

We need stricter laws governing wrong doers when they are our employers. It seems the laws regarding workers safety are being ignored. Safety violators and harassers are ruling the day. A person with a legitimate claim for a work related injury should not have to fight a system that is in the wrong. Obama said before he was elected that he would work on correcting the fact that disabled people have not been able to get their disability insurance for the past two decades.

We have had this kind of behavior from the judicial system and politicians for far too long. Too many times claims are pushed to the court level and the injured parties lose when they can't afford to pay for lawyers and court fees. Governor Strickland said when he was in office, we need a one stop shop in Ohio on heavy metals, but this is obviously not what happens! It is the responsibility of a president to preside over the judicial system and to overturn a judge's authority when they have made a mistake in judgment and not followed the laws of the land. The Supreme Court Laws should take precedence in this case.

We need reform in toxic tort laws as well as worker's comp laws. No one should lose their health, become disabled and have to try to live on social security alone. I have learned that self insured employers are not governed by ERISA laws. This means that they can determine how they want to administer their long term disability policies. This needs to definitely change. They should either be governed by the same laws every one else is governed by or lose their right to be self insured. The problem has been that people aren't aware of how the system works unless they have become a victim of it.

Too many injured people become totally disabled because their physical therapy is delayed. My workers comp lawyer said, "Everyone I know that ends up on workers comp becomes totally disabled." He also stated, "it isn't politically correct to be on the side of the worker in workers comp cases." This was the first time I talked with him. I was taken back and didn't understand what he meant by saying this. Now I know what he meant.

As I stated earlier the mitochondria have been found to be damaged in CF/FM. This comes with free radical damage and toxins. Check out the Montague Hooper Paper from 2001. They have identified an enzyme that becomes damaged and can not take out viruses like it should. They indicate this happens with toxins this no doubt is the root cause of chronic fatigue syndrome.

CELLULAR DAMAGE IN CHRONIC FATIGUE/FIBROMYALGIA

There was a good article in the Fibromyalgia Network newsletter of April 1994. Dr. S. Jacobsen, M.D. of Sweden reported that a subgroup of FMS patients had low levels of pro-collagen peptide in their blood. This he wrote is a particular peptide byproduct of collagen synthesis. Collagen is the building block for connective tissue used throughout the body to support muscles, ligaments and tendons. Dr. Jacobsen found that severity of symptoms correlated with lower than normal collagen synthesis. Remember earlier I mentioned that growth hormone is thought to control collagen synthesis. Wouldn't it then follow that by supporting the growth hormone or collagen in the body you might turn this problem around? I believe this is probably a result of poor nutrient assimilation due to the leaky gut syndrome.

You might ask for a Bio 101 test which looks at mineral and digestive assimilation. You might find that you aren't breaking down carbs or proteins. You may have enough digestive power but just are not absorbing the nutrients. In my case I had low levels of protein and minerals so I was told to take digestive enzymes with every meal. I have learned that we need proteolytic digestive enzymes (pancreatic enzymes) to break foods down. There are a lot of enzyme formulas on the market but you may also need the proteolytic enzymes if you are not producing enough enzymes to break down you're foods.

The other damage that has become obvious in CF/FM is the damage to the mitochondria of the cells. When the mitochondria become damaged they can't produce energy within the cells this can lead to energy crashes and severe fatigue. There are many products on the market now to address this problem, but if the internal landscape is littered with toxic chemicals and metals you will not get well. You will have to address the methylation system. Remember metals damage the P450 enzyme that helps the liver detox. There may also be other enzymes in the liver detox pathway that become damaged. See archived articles on liver toxicity. There are blood tests for the P450 enzyme.

I hope to give you some good direction to find the underlying problem and not just address the symptoms of your condition. I was just reading that visits to the ER for severe muscle pain and fatigue are sky rocketing. With all the pollution in the environment is it any wonder we have cellular damage to our bodies.

There is a new site called "We the People" where you can find petitions to our government. There are many important issues here! I have been watching the petitions on labor laws and find it curious that they don't seem to stay out there very long. They have raised the number of votes needed to 20,000 from 5,000. When you vote you might receive comments back from the white house on how you voted on some of the petitions. I thought the objective of the sight was to be heard but it doesn't seem to be working out that way.

One that I favor is the one asking them to Enforce Labor Laws and to protect injured workers that report safety violations from retaliation from employers. There was a law recently passed to protect OSHA whisleblowers. When an employee reports a serious safety violation it protects them from retaliation. We need to be vigilant to see that these laws that protect workers are enforced. Too many have lost their rights, their health and their way of life! You can find information on the welding rod cases in Cuyahoga County, Cleveland Ohio. They have only approved one case that I am aware of this was due to the injured person developing Parkinson's from welding. I know first hand the damage metals can do to the endocrine, neurological and immune systems.

Justice Frances Sweeney of Ohio's Supreme Court wrote "To deny an employee the right to file an action before he or she discovers that the injury was caused by the employer's wrongful conduct is to deny the employee the right to bring any claim at all."

When Strickland was governor he stated, "We need a one stop shop for heavy metals." I wrote him to say many people who work in industrial settings are being exposed to heavy metals not just the workers exposed to welding rod injuries. Their claims are being blocked. When I last studied this issue there was only one claim allowed because the person developed Parkinson's disease. Obviously the scientific literature is full of health issues related to heavy metal exposures. You don't have to look far to find it. Even the CDC and OSHA acknowledge these issues, so why are the claims for these injuries being blocked by the Industrial Commission of Ohio, and I wonder how many other states?

I don't think it takes a genius to figure the answer to this problem. Special interest seems to take precedence over the rights of injured workers.

The promise to the people has been broken for too long. Too many able bodied persons are disabled by their inability to get the appropriate and prompt care that they need. A short sighted view of a long term problem is causing a burden on all the citizen's of this nation. Some disabilities might have been avoided had the physical therapy been given and surgeries been avoided or the proper diagnosis been rendered.

No one wants to lose their health and become a statistic or have to live a meager existence and struggle to pay for care they can't afford. Care that should have been covered by the entities that caused their long term disability in the first place. An even worse scenario is someone who can't afford any care they have to pay for out of pocket, which is many times the case in any alternative care such as chelation therapy.

The Bible has something to say about governments that oppress and harm the people. It says the heads of state that caused harm to the people will have the harshest judgment when God returns to judge. It states, "It would have been better for them to have had rocks tied around their feet and dumped in the middle of the ocean." They will be the first to be judged and the harshest judgment will be dealt to them. They might want to consider this when they deny a person their right to a legitimate claim for injury and disability. Of course we have had special interest groups who have tried to take God out of our government and out of our schools. Could the natural disasters we are seeing be coming as a judgment for turning our backs on God? Many think this is the reason for the things taking place. The prophecies are being fulfilled daily; you only have to read your bible to know this is a fact. One thing being disabled has allowed me to do is spend time with the Lord. I have been blessed by this; his word has opened my eyes to what is going on!

The Montague Hooper Paper of 2001

The Montague Hooper Paper of 2001 reported that they had found the enzyme designed to take our viruses becomes damaged and this shows up as low 37 kDa sized enzyme produced by calpain (an apoptotic enzyme) the whole process affects the calcium and potassium channel mechanism. A higher ratio of 37 kDa and 80 KDa enzymes is associated with more severe clinical symptoms in CFS.

Both abnormal RNaseL activity and low oxygen consumption were observed in most patients with CFS. Low tolerance for physical activity may be linked to poor oxygen transport by red blood cells due to free radical damage. The mitochondria of the cells also can become damaged by free radical activity. This prevents the process of converting proteins and sugars into energy within the cells.

Increased apoptosis (programmed cell death in peripheral blood monuclear cells) has been suggested to contribute to the symptomology of CFS.

Baseline heart rate and plasma epinephrine were increased in CFS patients suggesting an activated sympatho-adrenal state. Sympathetic nervous system dysfunction is integral to CFS pathology.

Eighty five studies confirm autonomic nervous system dysfunction in 90% of CFS patients. This can result in changes of (blood pressure, pulse rate, breathing and body temperature). Substantial evidence that both the sympathetic and parasympathetic nervous system are abnormal in CFS.

When you experience visual changes, it is an indication that the connective tissue turnover time has been altered. This could be associated with low growth hormone and low collegen production.

There is evidence of a degenerative process of muscle tissue in CFS as occurs in myopathies. This may contribute to muscle fatigability and it supports an organic origin for CFS.

One virus which is known to activate the coagulation system is the HHV-6. I'm sure others may be capable of triggering the same response as the immune system becomes activated.

Environmental influences which researchers worldwide are investigating include the frequent pairing of CFS with food and chemical sensitivities.

The RNaseL pathway is a series of enzymatic reactions which go on inside white blood cells when they perceive themselves to be challenged by viruses and possibly also by some toxic exposures.

CHRONIC FATIGUE FIBROMYALGIA WRONG DIAGNOSIS

I started searching for information on methylation blocks because I was having trouble with chelation therapy. What I found was eye opening!

These are excerpts from Richard A. Van Konynenburg, Ph.D.

Instead of using methylcobalamin this physician recommends using hydroxocobalamin a form of B-12. Some people can have down regulation in their detoxification pathways which make it harder to use the methylcobalamin.

A research paper by Dr. S. Jill James, Ph.D. found a connection between the methylation cycle block and glutathione depletion in autism. In my opinion, some people with polymorphisms (these are changes in genes) may do better with reduced glutathione rather than glutathione in its regular form. This was my experience. Just because someone has a gene for lets say high blood pressure does not mean he will develop it with proper diet. It does mean he may be at a higher risk to develop it if he eats a diet high in saturated fats or Trans fats or has other risk factors. I believe life style and diet have more impact on our health than genes. There was a show on TV that featured a fellow with severe heart disease. He totally got rid of his heart disease by switching to a vegetarian live food diet. Of course this didn't happen over night; he had to stay on this protocol for months. The fact that he was scheduled for quadruple bypass surgery before starting this protocol speaks volumes!

Identified methylation cycle blocks and glutathione depletion in autism and chronic fatigue should be addressed before attempting to chelate heavy metals from the body in my opinion. Remember metals can damage the P450 enzyme pathway in the liver this might throw off the detox pathways of the liver as was my experience. Also it would be wise to correct nutrient deficiencies common in people with heavy metal toxicity. Without certain nutrients like B-12, B-6, zink, and folic acid, you may make the patient's situation worse by stirring up too many toxins that the body does not have the ability to get rid of itself.

My physician says he now checks everyone for nutritional deficiencies and blocks to the mehtylation system before attempting to chelate them. He stated that he had too many patients like me coming from other physicians who hadn't done well with the chelation.

We need to push to have insurances pay for these tests: as well as chelation therapy when it is needed, which are very important in finding the path back to health! Please write your senators!

You can find the full article at:

http://aboutmecfs.org/Trt/TrtGSHMeth1Simple.aspx

There were proposed rule-making for CFIDS/FM on social security many years ago.

Here is what was proposed in rule 58FR67574. Many people have probably not been aware of what social security looks at when they are deciding a case of disability for chronic fatigue/fibromyalgia.

This site stated that FM is caused by:

Disorders may result from heredity congenital, or acquired pathological processes. Impairments may result from infections, inflammatory or degenerative processes traumatic or developmental events or neoplastic, vascular or toxic metabolic diseases (these could come from chemical and metal toxicity).

Loss of function may be due to:

Bone or joint deformity or destruction from any cause, miscellaneous disorders of the spin with or without radiculopathy, or other neurological deficits, amputation, or fractures or soft tissue injuries.

Immune System

Specific diagnostic features that should be documented in the clinical record for each of the disorders are summarized for systemic lupus erythematosus (SLE) systemic vasculitis, systemic sclerosis & scleroderma, polymyositis connective tissue disorders, and the inflammatory arthritides.

Insurers have been known to put conflicting medical opinions in your files. If you are dealing with a long term disability insurer you can ask for your case records. It is a good thing to do to be sure they aren't putting in opinions that are counter to your medical records. You just have to send them a letter requesting these records. If they don't respond, you can consult your state representative for help.

They believe that some people are genetically predisposed to be more reactive to chemicals and heavy metals. I'm not aware that there are any genetic causes that have been proven.

Don't give up just keep looking for the root cause of your problems. I hope that I have given enough information in this book to help you do just that!

Health is our most valuable asset, do not let anything compromise it. Once it is gone you may have a hard time getting it back if it ever does come back.

Fibromyalgia/Chronic Fatigue and Toxic Liver

Do you have any of the following symptoms? Have you been on many medications? Could you have been exposed to chemical or metal toxins?

1) Low Energy?
2) Occasional Indigestion, Bloating, Diarrhea or Constipation?
3) Foggy Thinking?
4) Weight Gain/water retention?
5) Stiff, Aching, Weak Muscles?
6) Worries over Cholesterol?
7) Dealing with leaky gut syndrome?
7) Concerns about blood sugar—the liver stores sugar overnight so eating past dinner time might elevate sugar in the morning!

You might want to have a caffeine liver challenge test to see if you have an imbalance in the liver detoxification pathways. If you're regular M.D. is not familiar with this you might want to seek out a holistic practitioner who is also an M.D. They usually are familiar with this test. You can also have a blood test to check on the methylation system if something has affected the liver, you may not be able to effectively process and eliminate toxins. Metals can affect the P450 enzyme. This can also be tested.

Genetic testing may reveal that you have some polymorphisms that they believe can make it more difficult for you to get rid of toxins. The Genova Diagnostics is looking at these issues through gene testing. There have been differing opinions on this since some have not addressed the genes and simply supplemented the detox pathways. When they did this they did see improvement with these people. Until the damage to the mitochondria is addressed, even supplementing the detox pathway may not solve your fatigue and pain. I believe the whole key to eventually getting well is to heal the damage to the mitochondria. For those who have had long standing fibromyalgia, the damage in the muscle tissue and nervous system may not go away.

If you have damage to the liver and brain of course these are additional issues to be addressed. My physician believes you address the damage to the pituitary adrenal axis by supplementing 5-htp.

Check out These Sites:

http://www.gdx.net
http://www.thefibromyalgiadigest.com
http://www.freelupusdigest.com
If the liver is toxic nothing else will be right!

EXOGENOUS TOXINS AND CHRONIC FATIGUE SYNDROME

What are exogenous toxins? They are primarily products of the petrochemical industrial age. Industry has brought with it a high exposure to toxic heavy metals, namely aluminum, antimony, arsenic, beryllium, bismuth, cadmium, lead, mercury, nickel, platinum, silver, thallium, thorium, tin, and uranium. Before the industrial age we had little exposure to these elements other than silver and lead. When these elements enter the body they replace the nutritional elements of manganese and magnesium, etc. in enzyme systems. This means that enzymes that carry magnesium for example may be bound up by lead etc. You may be eating a healthy diet but the cells are starving for nutrients.

Other toxins are halogens such as chlorine and fluoride. These take the place of iodine on the receptor sites of cells thus blocking the absorption of Iodine according to Dr. David Brownstein who wrote the book on Iodine deficiency. No wonder we have a crisis of thyroid disease in this country!

Selenium is another nutrient that we are very deficient in because it has been depleted from the soil by modern farming using so many chemicals.

From the 1890s until the 1940s, organic chemicals were produced by the fractional distillation of coal and tar. No new chemicals were produced. In the 1940s using new technology, synthetic chemicals were created. It became possible to use petroleum to create new chemicals. In 1940 about one billion pounds of new synthetic chemicals were produced. By 1950, it had reached 50 billion pounds, and by the late 1980s it became 500 billion.

Water conducts any chemical or element it comes in contact with. No wonder they are finding new chemicals in our water supplies today. In areas where people engage in water sports and boaters paint the hulls with a paint to keep off barnacles; it has been found that a chemical is released from this paint and gets into the water supply. You may be at risk if your water comes from a reservoir where boating is allowed. Also boaters usually wash down their boats with caustic chemicals. They may also dump things into the water that really should not be there.

Of course chemicals that we use to keep down weeds in our yards and pesticides we spray around the outside of our homes can also be toxic substances. These eventually find there way into our waterways as well as the pesticides on farm lands and smoke stacks from manufacturing facilities.

If you are not concerned with the chemicals in your water you should be. Exogenous toxins have been found in areas where they fractionate the rock to get at gas deposits deep in the ground. They use water mixed with exogenous toxins and high pressure to break up the rock so they can drill down to get at the gas deposits. Many people may have therefore been exposed to these exogenous toxins without knowing it. This aired on one of the major news programs. Using carbon filters at the tap will help get rid of these exogenous toxins. Some of the states most affected were Ohio, Michigan and Pennsylvania. I just read on facebook that Wyoming has now been affected by contamination to underground water sources.

Lead is one exogenous toxin that can cause pain in the muscles, joints and tendons. It is known for causing auto-immune conditions in the body. It can be stored in the bones and soft tissues for 30 years and re-emerge when a person is under stress, trauma or has a change in their metabolic process such as developing the leaky gut syndrome. Recent research has linked M.S. to lead exposure.

There needs to me more research into the effects of these exogenous toxins and with more people being exposed doctors need to be more aware of the signs and symptoms of these exposures.

CHEMICAL INTOLERANCES AND CF/FM

I found a good article on chemical sensitivity in CF/FM at the www.imunesupport.com Web site.

The author wrote "I have noticed that many patients with fibromyalgia do not initially react to a new medication; that is, one tablet causes little or no response, the second tablet causes some response, and the third tablet might cause a violent reaction." I have experienced this myself.

They state, "These situations almost always coincide with the rapid decline of relaxin in the body". Relaxin affects the integrity of collagen, which makes up the mucosa, which acts as a sieve to filter nutrients. "I believe that mucosa integrity is compromised by relaxin deficit, so that the mucosa may leak or shut down completely." Could this explain the mechanism in the "leaky gut syndrome"? Are chemicals in drugs and the environment to blame? What Dr. Scott Rigden says might indicate they are to blame. He says what causes leaky gut are drugs like cortisone, naprosyn, antibiotics, bacterias and heavy metals. He was named researcher of the year two years ago. Dr. Cheney who has also treated over 3,000 CF/FM patients says these people are loaded with all kinds of chemicals and metals and have to be detoxed to make progress. He says they also have to heal the leaky gut!

"I believe that mucosa integrity is compromised by relaxin deficit, so that the mucosa may leak or shut down completely." In healthy patients, the ability of the mucosa to filter nutrients stays constant. "For patients with fibromyalgia, the mucosa may a) shrink in size so that few or no nutrients are absorbed or, b) open so completely that protein molecules of middle or larger molecular weight improperly leak into the rest of the body." This "all or nothing" response, called dysautonomia, can affect other areas of the body besides the mucosa.

For years doctors denied there was such a thing as leaky gut. They said that the muscular wave in the small intestine was missing which allowed too many bacterias to remain in this area which might cause an immune system reaction. There are test for leaky gut so it has been proven that in deed the mucosa lining can leak toxins and bacteria in to the system. (See tests for leaky gut)

Healing the leaky gut might help calm the immune system reaction to antigens in the system. Remember Dr. Cheney stated that you have to detox these people before you will see results. If they are dealing with chemicals and toxins, these may have to be removed from the body before you see a significant improvement in the person's health.

This has been true for me. Getting rid of long standing metal exposures can be an uphill battle, especially if your not absorbing nutrients or your methylation system is not functioning correctly.

Doctors are only now learning how essential it is to have the nutrient deficiencies addressed and the detox system working before trying to chelate the metals from their patients. Not addressing these issues first can cause more harm than good, just ask me, I have had the experience!

CHEAP TRICKS FOR CHRONIC FATIGUE FIBROMYALGIA

If you have read Dr. Teitelbaum's book on fibromyalgia you will find he has a long list of supplements that he recommends. A person could become overwhelmed trying to do all the things people are recommending for these conditions.

The most important issue is the compromised thyroid and adrenals. This must be addressed in order to see any progress. The second thing that I think is important is to address any intestinal issues that might be present. A comprehensive stool analysis is the best way to approach this. If there is an overgrowth of yeast or bacteria this must be addressed. People with heavy metal issues may well have an overgrowth of yeast or unfriendly bacterias. Stress and certain medications can also disrupt the gut flora. The good strains of lactobacillus and bifidus can be very helpful but you must be careful with these if you're dealing with leaky gut. Adding anything that might elicit an immune system response may not be desirable until you know if you're dealing with leaky gut. If you are dealing with this, you will want to work on healing this first, and then add the probiotics. If this isn't brought under control nothing else you do will matter.

An Elisa Assay is helpful to identify food intolerances.

Seek a good doctor. If all your doctor knows to do is hand out anti-depressants he hasn't been educated about CF/FM.

The best doctors I have found are M.D.'s that have gone back to school for continuing education in the holistic health field or integrative medicine as I prefer it to be called.

The most knowledgeable doctors I've found on the internet are Dr. Paul Cheney, Dr. Zoltan P. Rona and Dr. Scott Rigden. Do a search on any one of these outstanding physicians and you will find a treasure trove of helpful and insightful information on CF/FM.

Some of the best products I have found are:

Acetyl-L-Carnatine which helps with energy in the cells, mental energy, memory, and learning.

Carnosine helps support muscles, brain, skin and heart.

Cinnamon plus helps healthy glucose, metabolism and weight.

Daily Balancer gives top liver support and detoxification.

Digestive helper helps improve digestion of food.

GI soother helps sooth the digestive tract and supports digestive health.

Immune plus is a lymph system and immune support.

Iosol iodine supports thyroid and body temperature.

Leptinal is good aid in weight management, leptin function and cholesterol metabolism booster.

Melatonin helps support sleep rhythms.

These can be ordered through Wellness Resources at: http://www.chronicfatiguefibromyalgiawrongdiagnosis.com

Oregano oil is a potent sinus health enhancer and has natural anti-bacterial properties. Some people with gut issues however may be a little sensitive to it so go easy if you may be dealing with this. Some people with gluten intolerance may not tolerate this at all.

Oil of peppermint is a great product for opening up the sinuses. A few drops can be placed in a bowl of steaming hot water. Breath in the vapors and you will find relief of a stuffy nose in a few seconds. I use it when I have sinus congestion or a cold. I put a couple drops right under the nostril and you will have relief in seconds! It is also helpful for painful muscles. It helps the circulation of the blood which relieves tight aching muscles.

You can also use the oregano oil or oil of lavender where you have pain in the body. This is good for fighting systemic yeast.

I have also read that by placing rosewood a few drops at a time in your bath can be helpful in fighting viruses and yeasts. Periwinkle is also great at fighting viruses. White tea, holy basil (make tea) and rose help stop inflammation.

Magnesium muscle mag helps support muscle function. Magnesium has been found to be low in most people dealing with fibromyalgia. Magnesium is involved in over 100 bodily metabolism functions and is depleted from the foods we eat today. Magnesium, iodine and selenium have been depleted from our foods due to the way they have been raised. Metals can also bind up magnesium and other nutrients.

Pantethine is helpful for energy, adrenal function and normalizing cholesterol levels.

Co Q-10 is essential to the body without adequate levels you could experience a heart attack. Many statin drugs deplete Co Q-10 so you need to supplement if you are taking one of these drugs.

Sulfur Plus helps with respiratory system, removing toxins and strengthens skin and hair.

Thyroid helper has helped me maintain my armour thyroid levels and keep my thyroid from getting worse.

The Health and Wellness company has a catalog they will send out to you if you order any of their products which has a list of recommended products for any particular issue such as high blood pressure, sluggish adrenals, cardio-health, high cholesterol etc. There product formulas are backed by research.

I highly recommend you try their products. You can learn more about them by visiting my blog at http://www.chronicfatiguefibromyalgiawrongdiagnosis.com

I came across some information on a natural heavy metal cleanse, I don't know how effective this is but I do know that it tastes great!

Here is the recipe:

Metal Cleanse:
1 Packed Cup Fresh Cilantro
6 Tbs. Olive Oil—Blend these together and add
1 Garlic l/2 Cup Almonds or Cashews
2 Tbs. Lemon Juice

Blend to Lumpy Paste

You can add a little hot water to thin it down. Eat with crackers or bread and enjoy!

Here is a Recipe for Allergy Prevention:

Licorice root (the herb) helps build up immunity to allergens.

Add 3 oz. of cut licorice root (available at health food stores) to 1 quart of water. Boil 10 minites in enamel or glass pot, strain into bottle. Take 1 tablespoon before each meal, every other day until you've taken the licorice root water for six days.

You might find it interesting that some chiropractors recommend using licorice root pills to address leaky gut issues. Licorice has been known to help the body fight allergies.

There are many helpful herbs to build the immune system. You can find a lot of helpful information by visiting your local health food store. They have books on holistic health aids which can be very beneficial.

Herbs to build the immune system:

Passion flower which has many strong Native American roots and contains natural monoamine oxidase inhibitors known to have antidepressant and anti-anxiety properties.

Aswagandha—aphrodisiac and mood stabilizing properties, acts in adaptogenic fashion when androgen levels are low, activating hypothalamic-pituitary-gondal axis to increase the production of androgens.

Ginseng—acts as an adaptogen, helps you deal with stress

Echinacea—Helps stimulate the immune response

POLITICAL ACTION

Remember our representatives don't have to worry about becoming disabled or losing their health they have voted themselves in permanent health care and pay even after they leave office. They are often on the side of business because they help them get elected. I believe pay raises and benefits should coincide with services rendered, just like workers earn raises according to service and merit. They should also receive a pension, not full salary after they leave office. Why should they be paid as if they are still working? Is there any job in the public sector that can vote themselves a permanent salary? Senator Rick Perry suggest we have a part time congress. I think it would serve the country more if they had jobs or go on pension after they leave office, not have full time pay!

We need to do away with lobbyist and special interest groups as well as corporation funded politicians. If we could eliminate funds from special interest groups and lobbyists, our elected officials might feel more compelled to represent the people they are suppose to be representing, the people of the United States of America the citizens.

President Obama said he wanted to stop big oil and pharmaceuticals from running America. How has he done that? He also stated we are all Americans able bodied, disabled, every nationality and creed. Then it is time we all had a voice in our government! He also said he wanted to correct the fact that disabled people had been denied their right to their insurance coverage for two decades. It is obvious that little has been done to address these issues.

I believe our founding fathers intended that the public office would be held by people who had the interest of the citizens at heart. This seems to have eroded away since we now have special interest and corporations that can destroy the welfare of the people. We only have to reflect on the fact that destroyed companies still paid CEO's large salaries while filing for bankruptcy. I personally know of two families who had their life's savings wiped out when GM went in and raided the stocks their employees placed with them. They only received pennies on the dollar for the stock they had purchased. After they had served this company for many years.

I also know of people who have paid in to long term disability policies only to find out they couldn't collect past the two year own occupation limits even when their physicians said they were permanently disabled. They can just say you can go do something else while ignoring what your doctors have written in your medical records. If you don't have the funds to fight this, you lose or maybe even worse you aren't told what is in the reports, or are mislead to believe your doctor isn't standing behind you as was my case. You may have to ask for the records to find out what your doctor is actually saying.

Recently Dr. Oz spoke about the fact that they now consider pain to be a disease in and of itself.

I found this interesting since my research shows they have known that pain that persists for hours every day leads to changes in the central nervous system. This was written about in the Fibromyalgia Network newsletter back in October 1996.

According to Ron Dubner, Ph.D., of the university of Maryland in Baltimore, stated "pain that persists for hours every day leads to changes in the central nervous system." "The changes result in amplification and increased sensation of pain." He stated this happens when the nerves at the level of the spinal cord are hit with a persistent barrage of pain signals from the body's peripheral tissues.

According to pain receptor researcher Dr. Frank Porreca, of the University of Az. in Tucson, 70% of your opioid receptors are located in the periphery organs, muscles and other issues, or at the level of the spinal cord juncture before entering the dorsal horn. Only 30% are located in the dorsal horn and brain. This is important to keep in mind, because under acute pain situations, opiates like morphine and codeine will work on those opioid receptors in the periphery to reduce the pain.

To better understand why chronic pain syndromes like FMS are not the same as an acute pain situation, you have to know a little bit about how your body is supposed to deal with pain signals coming from the periphery, such as muscles, soft tissues and organs. Many of the repetitive sensory stimuli healthy people receive on a daily basis are either filtered out or down-regulated in importance at the level of the dorsal horn by neurotransmitters released in this area to control pain.

Substances like serotonin and norepinephrine act as opioids under a normal situation, while cholecystokinin works to block opioids and increase pain. Some of the signals may reach the thalamus, the caudate nuclei and the limbic system can send inhibitory messages back down to the dorsal horn to reduce pain.

They know the substance "P" which is a pain conducting chemical becomes elevated in people with FM. Other substances like EAAs and DGRP in the brain that cause perception of pain may also be elevated making someone with fibromyalgia more sensitized to pain signals from the body.

If you have read the advertisements for the drug "Lyrica" they state that fibromyalgia is thought to be a condition of overactive nerves in the muscle tissues. Lyrica was designed to calm the nerves but the side affects I have read say it can lead to muscle aches and weakness. Those of us with fibromyalgia already have painful and achy muscles, why would you take something that could add to this problem? I have read some comments about people with these conditions who have had some pretty nasty side affects from using this drug. Why not look for the underlying cause of the muscle and nerve conditions?

Do a search on Dr. Paul Cheney "Leaky Gut Syndrome" or Dr. Scott Rigden "Leaky gut syndrome!" You might also check with Dr. Zoltan P. Rona. He seemed to know about leaky gut before any of our physicians in the U.S. Of course there were doctors writing opinions that there was no such thing as leaky gut when I was diagnosed. They said we had just lost the wave in the small intestine that removes bacterias! I think the real reason for the denial of leaky gut for so long goes to the issues that cause it!

IMMUNE ABNORMALITIES IN CHRONIC FATIGUE SYNDROME

I talked earlier in an article on leaky gut syndrome about how proteins enter the bloodstream through a bowel that has become hyper-permeable. If you look at my information on metabolic origin, you will find they mention high pyruvates in the blood. How does this happen? Pyruvates occur because of an abnormal carbohydrate metabolism. In other words you may not be producing enough amylase enzymes from the pancreas to break down carbohydrates. You may also be dealing with leaky gut syndrome.

Drugs and heavy metals can affect the digestive system. Metals also block the enzymes necessary to carry nutrition to the cells. This is why metals lead to a weakened muscle skeletal system. This is being studied and recently stated the higher the exposure the more muscle skeletal problems will occur.

High levels of glycation end product modified proteins (AGE) are produced when there is a hyper-permeable state of the intestines. Glycogens (sugars) and proteins can cross link in the muscle fibers forming small band like structures that can cement the muscle fibers together. This causes muscle tissue damage. The AGE induced tissue damage occurs once the antioxidant reserves of the muscle are used up. This damage activates excess production of NF-kappaB which contributes to the muscle pain and perpetuates the damage. As the problem continues the antioxidant defense system is used up. At this point, excess NF-kappa B is activated in an inflammatory manner. This causes a progression of local tissue damage and results in excess pain. The nerves may also be involved. This process also happens with age and onset of diabetes.

The longer a person stays in FM pain, the more likely it is that damage is done to the muscles.

When under stress most people with fibromyalgia will experience a flair or exacerbation of their muscle pain. I always wondered why this was and just recently learned that when corticotropin releasing hormone from the hypothalamus gland is released from the brain it initiates the stress response. When this hormone was injected into FM patients it stayed elevated in the blood whereas levels should return to normal in someone not suffering with fibromyalgia. This reflects a general hormone resistance across the board in adapting to stress. This could explain how severe stress and trauma leads into fibromyalgia. It also explains why stress makes fibromyalgia pain worse.

Leptin is the master hormone of the body that has many functions besides controlling weight gain or weight loss. In fibromyalgia the hypothalamus may lose control over the adrenals and other hormone functions such as leptin.

To learn more about getting leptin back in to proper functioning you may want to order Bryan Richards book "Mastering Leptin" he has a chapter on fibromyalgia and his insight helped save me when I began losing weight and was in an anorexic weight loss syndrome which I could not seem to control. Obviously my leptin hormone must have been practically non existent. Sometimes people experience this before they die, when they are very ill, or they have lost control of the cortisol response from the adrenals.

I followed his suggestions along with taking "Boost" etc. and it turned my situation around in about three weeks. Thanks Bryan you may have saved my life! I never came across anyone who understood the underlying metabolic process like Bryan Richards. His book is full of nuggets of wisdom and it isn't very expensive! You can find it by clicking on "Health Resources" in the upper right hand corner of my web blog:

http://www.chronicfatiguefibromyalgiawrongdiagnosis.com

Nerve pain is the result of a worn down nervous system. When someone has had fibromyalgia for a long time they may experience pain in the nerves even from thinking of something that is pleasant. Any amount of emotion that can send energy through the nervous system, can be felt as pain. Nerves can also be injured in the process of an overactive immune system that produces antibodies which can attack the myelin sheath around the nerves as occurs in M.S. and auto-immune reactions weather from exposure to metals or chemicals. I found a research article that said when lead gets stirred up in the blood it can cause M.S. because it sends the immune system in to an over-active state. Is it any wonder people with toxin exposures are experiencing stress on the body. Cytokines are produced in response to these toxins. Cytokines set off the inflammatory response!

When stress is ongoing a person enters a phase of excess sympathetic nerve activity or surplus adrenaline. This leads to adrenaline resistance, insulin resistance, and leptin resistance. Leptin resistance can cause weight gain and also weight loss as in an anorexic metabolism.

Elaine Marie Graham

CHRONIC FATIGUE

NK levels and function per cell (not just gross killing) is mandatory as is measurement of the CD4-CD8 ratio; other immunologist tests should include testing for ANA's (anti-nuclear antibodies) IgG's including IgG3 CIC (circulating immune complexes) IL2; IL4 (interleukin 2 & 4) measurement of Th1-Th2 response and mitogen stimulation tests.

Test for thyroid antibodies:
Natelson el al—demonstrated link between IL4 and a type 2 cytokine pattern in ME/CFS a preponderance of a Th2 response is consistent with autoimmunity.

Antilamen antibodies in ME/CFS (antibodies against this protein are proof of autoimmunity and of damage to brain cells). 52% of ME/CFS patients develop auto antibodies to components of the nuclear envelope (NE) hormonal autoimmunity against polypeptides of the NE is a prominent immune derangement.

Auto antibodies to an intracellular protein like lamin B1 provides lab evidence for an autoimmune component in ME/CFS No patients with depression showed reactivity to NE proteins.

Auto antibodies to NE proteins are relatively infrequent in routine ANA serology and most of these fall into the broad category of an unusual connective tissue disease subset which is characterized by brain or skin vasculits.

Auto antibodies to a cellular protein expressed primarily in ME/CFS patients in neuronal cells (MAP2). Immunohisto-chemistry results showed a high reactivity in ME/CFS patients as also in patients diagnosed with lupus and rheumatoid arthritis.

OTHER CONDITIONS RELEATED TO CF

Coxsackie B virus has been found in cardiac, pancreatic gut dysfunction.

Endocrine—adrenals reduced by 50% in chronic fatigue patients.

Testing for Rombergism and nystagmus of all nervous systems in ME/CFS mandatory often overlooked!

Test for sympathetic over-activity and orthostatic hypotension should be done.

Hypofusion of brain stem—brain perfusion impairment provides evidence of central nervous system dysfunction.

Oxidative metabolism—is reduced

Lung function—is reduced

Hypercoagulability—fibrinogen, prothrombin fragment 1 & 2 thrombin/anti-thrombin, soluble fibrin monomer and platelet activation by flow cytometry)

Evidence of a degenerative process of the muscle tissue in CFS patients as typically occurs in mitochondrial myopathies. This may contribute to muscle fatigability—supports organic origin for CFS.

Researchers in Norway have published some very promising results of a controlled clinical trial of rituximab, a biologic agent used to treat certain cancers and rheumatoid arthritis. Two thirds of patients improved after two infusions.

Here is a link to more info. www.cfids.org/catalyst2011.pdf

SYMPTOMS OF CHRONIC
FATIGUE SYNDROME/FM

1) Shortness of breath upon exertion
2) Ice pick like pains or electrical pain that shoots into a muscle, hand or foot
3) Nosebleeds
4) Metallic taste or other unnatural taste in the mouth
5) Vertigo, dizziness
6) Ringing in ears (tinnitus)
7) Rage or inappropriate anger
8) Panic attack or anxiety
9) Depression
10) Tingling needles and pins sensation
11) Increased sensitivity to touch
12) Difficulty with sleep, staying asleep and getting to sleep
13) Mood Swings
14) Excessive thirst Frequent Urination
15) Impotence
16) Irregular Vaginal Bleeding
17) Low body temperature
18) Chronic yeast infections (metals suppress immune system)
19) Onset of menopause (imbalance in hormones)
20) Muscle aches and pains

21) Headaches
22) Visual changes (difficulty with fluorescent lighting or bring lights)
23) Blood pressure changes
24) Digestive system disturbances (irritable bowel syndrome)
25) Food intolerances
26) Leaky gut syndrome

It was found the urinary creatine test done on people with ME/CFS excreted significant levels of creatine and other muscle related metabolites including choline and glycine. This may represent ongoing muscle damage. Creatine has previously been shown to be a sensitive marker of muscle inflammation.

There is also evidence of hypercoagulability in ME/CFS. There is also evidence of dysfunction in the sympathetic and parasympathetic nervous systems.

When there is a link between IL4 and type 2 cytokine pattern a preponderance of a Th2 response is consistent with autoimmunity.

It was found that the RNase L pathway enzyme was elevated in the beginning of developing CFS. Expression of low molecular weight RNase L can cause problems with enzymatic detoxification pathways particularly in the liver.

Professor Vojdoni and Dr. Charles Lapp, found this same antiviral pathway can be damaged by chemicals. This is why it is so important to avoid them as much as possible. Dr. Howard Unovitz from the Chronic Journal of the American Society for microbiology and in Clinical Microbiology Review has demonstrated a fundamental linking of toxic exposure with chronic diseases such as ME/CFS and other autoimmune disorders.

A large number of CFS patients have an abnormal immunological profile which can result in the production of immunologic mediators such as interferon, interleukin and the cytokines. This might indicate chemical and metal exposures are contributing to this response as well as intolerances to foods.

RISK FACTORS FOR DEVELOPMENT OF CF/FM

1) Physical trauma or surgery
2) Chemical Exposure to toxins (heavy metals), organophosphates, pesticides, solvents
3) Biological infections, vaccines, blood transfusions, insect bits, allergic reactions
4) Poor quality sleep due to pain etc.
5) Emotional turmoil or long standing stress
6) Psychological issues stemming from stress or chronic pain syndromes

Stressors cause demands on cortisol production from the adrenal glands. This also depletes the production of epinephrine and nor epinephrine and goes on to eventually deplete the production of glutathione. This is important because glutathione is our master antioxidant that is produced in the liver and blood cells. Glutathione helps rid the body of toxins. If glutathione becomes depleted, the toxins can build up in the body tissues and glands. Glutathione can also be bound up by mercury. I believe as toxins build in the tissues glutathione is then further depleted. Also issues of leaky gut would put a huge demand on the body's detoxification and immune systems as the immune system has to mount a defense to rid itself of antigens in the blood that should not be there.

It was first suggested by Note and Droge and Holm that glutathione was depleted in ME/CFS back in 1997. Dr. Cheney also noted reduced glutathione in his patients.

It has been found that glutathione also supports phase I and II of the liver detox systems.

It was found that people with CF/FM had low glutathione, low B-12 and deficiencies in their methylation system. They also could have low folate and nutritional deficiencies when dealing with metals.

GLUTATIONE DEPLETION IS LINKED TO THE FOLLOWING:

1) Oxidative Stress
2) Mitochondrial dysfunction
3) Build up of toxins and heavy metals
4) Immune dysfunction
5) Herpes viruses
6) Thyroid problems
7) Deregulation of Cysteine
8) Low and dysregulated ACTH leading to blunted HHPA axes. Low anti-diuretic leads to high daily urine volume and low cortisol

9) Perforin which takes out mutant cells becomes low due to low glutathione and problems in the methylation cycle

10) These issues can lead to an over expression of genes because of lack of gene silencing by methylation system. The methylation system involves the liver

GLUTATHIONE IS MADE FROM THREE AMINO ACIDS, GLYCINE, CYSTEINE, AND GLUTAMIC ACID OR GLUTAMINE

Glutamine is found in protein foods, such as beans, fish, chicken, and eggs as well as in vegetables such as cabbage, spinach, beets, and tomatoes.

Cysteine is a sulfur-containing amino acid found in onions, garlic, and eggs.

Glycine is found plentifully in root vegetables and sprouts.

By getting plenty of these amino acids you will be getting the building blocks for glutathione.

LIVER DETOXIFICATION REQUIRES SPECIAL NUTRIENTS

N-acetylcysteine found in onions and garlic

Coenzyme Q10, found in oily fish, spinach, and raw seeds and nuts

Vitamin C, found in broccoli, peppers, citrus fruits, and berries

Vitamin E, found in raw seeds, nuts, and fish

Selenium, found in raw seeds, nuts, and fish

Beta-carotene, found in carrots, peaches, watermelon, sweet potatoes, and butternut squash

You can detoxify excess estrogens and chemicals like PCBs and dioxins, herbicides and pesticides with cruciferous vegetables such as broccoli.

PROTECT THE LIVER;

Bioflavonoids such as antocyanidins in blueberries, quercetin in red onions, polypehnols in green tea, and the herb milk thistle.

PHASE II OF THE LIVER DETOX SYSTEM;

I just recently came across a company that is producing a product that supplies the nourishment to boost the production of glutathione within the cells. They have many patents on their Cellgevity product. We spoke with one of their distributors and she was very interesting. She says that there is one physician who is traveling the country to do seminars on their products. He had such great results with his own patients he wanted to tell the world about his experience with them.

My husband and I noticed that we were experiencing results with the Cellgevity product the first day we took them. This is remarkable since supplementation usually takes some time before you see any results. We are excited about this company and the impact which we feel will be very positive on anyone's health who decides to give these products a try. We have had an increase in stamina and a decrease in fatigue.

You can find the products for Max International products at the following web site:
http://www.max.com/359989

People with Higher Glutathione Levels:

Have more Energy
Recover Faster From Exercise
Sleep Better
Have Greater Mental Clarity and Focus
Less Inflammation
Improved Joint Function
Have Better Immune Systems
Live Longer
Live Better
Improve the Health and Function of Every Cell, Tissue and Organ in the Body.

Glutathione has the ability to neutralize many types of free radicals that assault the cells. It is the only antioxidant that recycles itself again and again to continue fighting free radicals.

Glutathione is:

A powerful Chelator of Heavy Metals
Protects Immune Cells
Protector of Mitochondria DNA. The lower the glutathione level, the more vulnerable this DNA becomes to breakages.
Protects Nucleus of the Cell
Reduces Oxidative Stress

Reduces Intercellular Inflammation
Reducing Agent for Hemoglobin, allowing it to transport oxygen to every cell.

Environmental toxins will deplete the glutathione levels within the body. Your glutathione is decreasing, but the attacks on your cells are not! I just can't say enough about the great benefits of raising your glutathione levels. Low glutathione levels have been linked to 74 different disease processes some of which are the ones we worry about the most! Raising the glutathione will help with the livers detox pathways! Glucuoronidation is the most important detoxification pathway and it depends on calcium D-glucarate. (Lead will bind calcium so it is important to get rid of it)

Eat lots of apples, brussels sprouts, broccoli, cabbage, and bean sprouts to boost this pathway.

Sulfation:

Depends on the sulfur-containing amino acids found in onions, garlic, and eggs. You can also supplement MSM which helps the body detoxify.

Mehylation:

This key detoxifying process depends on B vitamins, especially folic acid (in greens and beans), vitamin B12 (animal souce only), and vitamin B6 as well as trymethylgycine (TMG), once again found in root vegetables.

DEFICIENCIES ASSOSCIATED WITH CHRONIC FATIGUE SYNDROME

1) Low Co Q 10
2) Lowered synthesis of carnatine
3) Lower synthesis of myelin
4) Low folate—causing rise in figlu
5) Low folate—low white cell count poor digestion
6) Metabolism of estrogen becomes a problem
7) Enzymes involved in estrogen detox—1B1 COMT SOD—super oxide demutase
8) Lack of ATP (energy production in cells)
9) Mitochondrial dysfunction—leading to chronic fatigue
10) Toxins build up in motochondria because of lack of glutathione
11) Exercise—causes oxidative reactive species (this is why it is criminal to expect someone with CF/FM to do aerobic exercise!) (See The Montague Hooper Paper of 2001)

The methylation process helps control gene expression, distributes CH3—bio reactions in body. Controls sulfur metabolism. Oxidative stress lowers cysteine, it also mutates DNA and leads to cancer. This is how I know it is a miracle I have not yet had cancer!

When glutathione is depleted, it causes problems in secretory protein synthesis.

The hypocampus can be damaged by high cortisol production when under prolonged stress in early part of the process which leads to developing CF/FM.

There are over 98,000 scientific studies and articles on glutathione recorded on Pub Med, the official U.S. Government library of medical research. There is a new supplement company that also has a patented product which doctors are now using in their medical practices and getting great results. This product is called Cellgevity by Max International. Glutathione can be reduced by metal toxins.

Could this explain the genesis of autism? How about CF/FM?

INFORMATION ON CF

The drug Rituxan which contains monoclonal antibodies was approved for two forms of cancer and rheumatoid arthritis and has also been given to CF patients.

There were published studies of immune abnormalities in a subset of CFS patients going back to the 1990s.

S boulardii is a new probiotic which they feel helps prevent antibiotic associated diarrhea and CDAD—clostridium difficile associated diarrhea. Researchers found that those with inflammatory bowel disease were four times more likely to develop neuromuscular conditions, including carpel tunnel and small fiber neuropathy which causes pain and lack of feeling in the feet.

Those with bowel disease are also 6 times more likely to have sensori-motor polyneuropathy, a nerve disease that can cause weakness pain and numbness.

Inflammatory bowel disease patients commonly also suffer from several other medical conditions like B-12 deficiency and glucose intolerance. These nerve conditions are often not diagnosed by their primary physicians. Rates of inflammatory bowel disease are rising in both adults and children. The major types are Cohn's disease and ulcerative colitis and symptoms can include pain, diarrhea, rectal bleeding and weight loss.

The U.S. government has announced a phase out of use of mercury amalgams.

They formally stated that "any change toward the use of dental amalgam is likely to result in positive public health outcomes." It will be interesting if the bowel problems go down along with this course of action!

DANGERS IN VACCINES WHAT DID THE CDC KNOW?

A federal case has been filed asking the CDC for information under the FOIA (Freedom of Information Act) to disclose what they have known about the dangers of mercury in vaccines. The case is Brian S. Hooker V. CDC. There is a move to shut down this information. It will be an interesting case to watch. You can follow its progress by going to Tim Bolen's consumer watch site on the internet. He keeps us up on what we need to know about cases which directly affect the health of the U.S. citizens. He has been following the "quackwatch" case for some time. The quackwatch group has tried to discredit physicians who use Doctor's Data Laboratories for their urine analysis of heavy metals. The quackwatch group lost a case in California and it was determined that they were "biased and unworthy of credibility." I was bowled over when my former employer brought this garbage into one of my worker's comp hearings and insinuated that all doctors doing chelation are on the fringe of medicine. It will be interesting to watch this group of quackwatchers go down in infamy. It is time injured people saw some justice in the judicial system!

DANGERS OF AN ACIDIC BODY PH

The pancreas can be harmed if the body is metabolically too acid because it tries to maintain bicarbonates. Without sufficient bicarbonates, the pancreas is slowly destroyed, insulin becomes a problem and hence diabetes becomes an issue.

In conjunction with this is the inability to produce enough bicarbonate essential for the production of pancreatic enzymes. The body's bicarbonate level remains fairly constant until age 45, and decreases about 18% by 90. Degenerative diseases start at around 45, this might be avoided if the body PH is maintained at a more alkaline level.

The lack of magnesium may contribute to an acidic PH. Without this nutrient the body accumulates toxins and acid residues, degenerates rapidly and ages prematurely.

In low selenium areas the number of people struck down by cancer is three times higher than in areas where selenium is more available in the soil.

THOUGHTS CONTROL GENES

It has been said that there are over 100 genes in the body that are turned on by thoughts, feelings and experiences. We can have a positive impact by taking control of our thoughts. Remembering one bad experience can lower the immune system production of antibodies for up to 6 hours. It is any wonder someone racked by pain and fatigue every day might have a problem controlling their thoughts? Negative thoughts produce stress hormones that might make the body more acidic.

Just like controlling thoughts, we have to control how many toxins we allow in to any degree possible. I have an environ care unit which filters toxins coming in from outside when the air circulates through the furnace system. I'm sure this cuts down on airborne particles that might get into our home. When I have cleaned it, it looks like coal dust is lining the rungs on the inside of the filters.

We believe reverse osmosis is the most effective method for filtering your water for drinking water in your home. We also have a whole house water softener unit since we have high levels of lime and minerals in our water here in Indiana.

TESTS FOR HEALTHY FOLKS TO CONSIDER

1) CRP which is a marker of inflammation in the body
2) Homocysteine—too much is a risk factor for a heart attack
3) Hemoglobin A1c for heart attack risk.
4) Hemoglobin Alc if diabetic
5) Early lung cancer and early CDT test
6) Vit. B12 (energy weight loss)

The CRP or C-reactive Protein if elevated indicates inflammation anywhere in the body. C-reactive protein is made in the liver and interacts with the complement system as part of your immune defense system. This protein can damage the endothelium and accelerates the progression of arterial artery plaque.

High blood homocysteine levels promote oxidation of lipids, platelet stickiness and the binding of an important fatty protein involved in clotting called lipoprotein to fibrin. Vitamins B-6, B-12, folic acid and trimethylglycine (TMG) are supplements proven to lower homocycsteine levels. It has been said homocysteine is the biggest contributor to heart disease.

Nattokinase which is a soy based enzyme is effective at dissolving the fibrin and thus reducing blood thickness and artherosclerosis which leads to heart disease and stroke.

B-12 deficiency has gone undetected in many cases and this can lead to heart attack and stroke. This deficiency can lead to damage to the myelin sheath that surrounds the nerves! This makes the nerves like frayed electrical wire making it harder for nerve cells to carry messages.

Victims can develop weakness, balance problems, leg and back pains, or glove and stocking numbness in hands and feet. It can also cause dizziness, vertigo or postural hyptertension (drop in blood pressure upon standing). In 2004 a study showed that there is a correlation between B-12 deficiency and osteoporosis! It can also lead to tremors handwriting difficulty and other symptoms severe enough to resemble early Parkinsons. Metals can bind up enzymes which carry nutrients to the cells leading to all kinds of nutrient deficiencies.

Nutrients which protect endothelium lining of blood vessels include folic acid, vitamin C, fish oil, alpha lipoic acid, (nutrients that suppress chronic inflammation.) It is possible to have near fatal deficiency of B-12 and still have normal lab test results.

You can test for methylmalonic acid in the urine. The test is the MMA test. Elevated levels indicate B-12 deficiency. The MMA/creatinine ratio test is the most accurate form of testing for B-12 deficiency.

Homocysteine test measures the level of homocysteine in the plasma. Elevated levels of homocysteine indicate B-12, B-6 or folate deficiency. The higher your HCY level, the higher your risk for cardiovascular disease!

It has been suggested that high levels of toxic homocysteine possibly stem from B-12 deficiency. This may cause microinfarcts which are tiny areas of blood vessel damage that trigger formation of plaques on tangles that eventually clutter the brain of a person with Alzheimer's. Low folate and B-12 along with elevated levels of homocysteine were associated with Alzheimer's disease.

Toxins like mercury can interfere with B-12 ability to cross the blood-brain barrier and reach neurons where it is needed. There can be a number of inborn errors of B-12 metabolism. Tests have shown low or no B-12 levels in the brains of people suffering with CFS,

Many problems can stem from B-12 deficiency which includes weakness, dizziness, nerve pain or numbness, mental illness, dementia or M.S. like symptoms, chronic fatigue, infertility or other medical problems.

Many doctors fail to diagnose people with B-12 deficiency, ascribing their symptoms to pre-existing conditions, other diseases, aging, heavy drinking, or mental illness and the result is catastrophic!

Tingling or pins and needles in hands and feet, memory loss, depression, personality changes, dizziness, loss of balance and outright dementia can all be related to B-12 deficiency. High levels of folate can make the complete blood count test appear normal even when B-12 deficiency exists.

Some reports suggest 15-20% of seniors have B-12 deficiency. Over 80% of vegans who do not supplement their diets with B-12 and over 50% of long term vegetarians show evidence of B-12 deficiency.

B-12 helps to clean toxins from tissues and organs, provide you with energy from food, protect against infection, repair damage, and allow your cells to communicate with each other.

A B-12 deficiency can hurt or kill you! If you have any of the mentioned symptoms, please get a test for this deficiency.

HELPFUL TIPS TO PREVENT THE FLU

1) Take Vitamin D and C daily.
2) Take 3 grams magnesium chloride 3 every 6-8 hrs helps combat the flu.
3) If you do get the flu you can put a clove of garlic in the blender, add 1/2 lemon, Add 6 oz. water and a pinch of cayenne—take this in the morning and before bed! I got rid of H1N1 and all congestion associated with it in just three days after starting on this remedy!

ROOT CAUSES OF INSOMNIA

1) Imbalances in stress hormones like cortisol or in neuro-transmitters like serotonin, Dopamine and GABA.
2) Too much stress! The herb Kava Kava is a great stress reliever and Valarian also helps with stress!

Melatonin taken l/2 hour before bed time works like a charm.

HEALTH WARNINGS!

It has been estimated that every year over 100,000 Americans are killed by drugs or drug interactions and it is estimated that two million are injured by drugs!

This is why I have leaned on the use of natural substances God created after being struck down with CF/FM and almost losing my life to the exposure of drugs and toxic metals. I am still dealing with the affects from the metals.

God knew when he made herbs and food that it was for our healing. I believe it is the exposure to chemicals and toxins which are causing reactions to our foods. The genetically modified grains also have 10 times the amount of gluten they had just 100 years ago. Gluten is hard to digest. I see advertisements for cereals now that state "now there are cereals I can give my children without having to worry." They are gluten free! Does anyone remember the recall on corn products because it was causing gut issues? I have read that Europe is outlawing genetically modified foods.

Who knows what the man made chemicals in drugs are doing to us, each person has their own genetic makeup, and there is no way to test to see what reaction they might have to any given drug. There are now severe reactions being seen to antibiotics which present as severe burns or allergic reactions. Some have died from these reactions, many have been hospitalized. There are new law suits daily for damages from drugs! Check out the Lawyers and Settlements site! They post these suits regularly.

Some other interesting sites to visit are:

Tim Bolen—health and consumer advocate http://www.bolenreport.com

Radio Liberty—Dr. Stan Monteith http://www.radioliberty.com

Prophecy in the News http://www.prophecyinthenews.com

Life Extension Foundation http://www.lef.org

Dr Russell Baylock Wellness Report http://www.baylockreport.com

Lawyers and Settlements http://www.lawyersandsettlements.com

The Jigsaw Health Website lists Holistic dentists and may direct you to help in getting your amalgam (silver) fillings removed from your mouth. Go to: http://www.jigsawhealth.org/

These sites will keep you abreast of what is going on in the world!

It has been said "All truth passes through three phases"

1) First it is ridiculed
2) It is violently opposed
3) Accepted as self evident

Author Thomas Keen

This reminds me of the denial that there was such a thing as leaky gut. They claimed you would be dead if this were the case. It has been proven, now there are laboratory tests for it and functional medicine has claimed it as the basis for chronic so called incurable diseases!

Will using chemo and radiation to kill cancer be next on the chopping block?

Will amalgams seem like an archaic medieval treatment for tooth decay?

Will autism spectrum syndrome be reversible? I believe it already is if treated early!

Will people's workers and human rights be restored?

Will mercury, aluminum and other irritants be removed from vaccines?

Will polluters be forced to clean up their environmental pollution?

Will civil rights be restored?

Will human rights be honored?

Will integrative treatments be accepted as standard medical practice?

Will insurance companies be held accountable or will they continue to be allowed to contribute heavily to the justice system and people in congress and continue policies as usual? Denying claimant's rights to their coverage under policies they paid into for years.

These are surely questions that beg to be answered! They will only be answered when the public demands an answer! We have to be the vanguards of our human and civil rights! These and other problems will only be resolved when we the people stand for what is right!

I had one physician tell me I would not get well until I forgave the people who exposed me to the heavy metals which lead to my disability. I said, "You can forgive someone and still hold them accountable for their actions can't you?" She said, "Yes I think you can do that." She then said, "You have righteous indignation and you have a right to have that just don't let it consume you." That is after all what the Lord does, he holds us accountable for our actions. We seem to have lost our moral fiber in this country. We have blurred the lines between what is right and what is wrong.

I have had to practice a lot of forgiveness by those who do not understand the conditions of CF/FM and how disabling they can be. I had one member of my family chide me with "everyone has some kind of pain Elaine." I wonder how well they would be doing if they were dealing with all the ramifications of these disorders. They have not understood my husbands fatigue over the years. Obviously anyone making such a statement really has no idea what someone else might be dealing with especially if they haven't studied the research on these disorders. My life has been an ongoing practice in forgiveness. I am however very convicted to get the research in the hands of people who need it and to keep pressing our lawmakers to do the right thing!

I had an expert witness who also testifies in toxic tort cases around the country look at my records. He said he would say in a court of law that my problems stemmed from these exposures. I also talked with a doctor who wrote the book on toxic exposures and he said he would also testify to this fact that the exposures caused my CF/FM. You can find his book on amazon, the title is "Toxic Tort" by Ernest P. Chiodo, M.D., J.D., M.P.H. C.I.H. If you are dealing with any toxic exposures, I recommend you get this book.

The Bible says, "I have provided all the herbs of the field and the leaves of the trees for your healing." The Bible also says, "Physician heal thyself." The body is always working on healing; we just have to remove the stumbling blocks to that healing by getting rid of toxins and eating a diet that will nourish the body! Hopefully you can do this before permanent damage sets in. A cleaner environment would surely go a long way in helping everyone reach these goals. Please write your congressmen and ask that they put scrubbers on the coal burning plants and manufacturers which produce pollutants. Please also ask that workers rights be restored and insurance policies be honored in a timely manor.

There is something in this book for everyone so please share it!

NEW GUIDELINES FOR OSHA WHISTLEBLOWERS

OSHA SARBANES-OXLEY ACT OF 2002 (SOX) from The Employeement Law Group Site!

On November 3, 2011, the Occupational Safety and Health Administration (OSHA) published interim final rules that modify regulations pertaining to whistleblower complaints filed under the Sarbanes-Oxley Act of 2002 (SOX). The Dodd-Frank Wall Street Reform and Consumer Protection Act of 2010 contained amendments that strengthen SOX whistleblower provisions. The recently released interim rules aim to bring SOX whistleblower regulations in line with the Dodd-Frank amendments and OSHA regulations for other whistleblower programs.

Broader protections for whistleblowers under Dodd-Frank Amendments

Significantly, Dodd-Frank extended protection for employees against workplace retaliation by credit rating agencies and other "nationally recognized statistical rating organizations" as defined in the Securities Exchange Act of 1934. 15 U.S.C. § 78c. The new OSHA rules adopt this definition and, similarly, modify the definition of "company" to mirror the definition under the Sarbanes-Oxley Act.

Extended complaint filing period and acceptance of oral complaints

Additionally, the regulations have been changed to reflect statutory changes to complaint filing procedures, extending the filing period for retaliation complaints under Sarbanes-

Oxley from 90 to 180 days after either the violation occurs or after the date on which the employee became aware of the violation. Most notably, the new rules clarify that oral complaints to OSHA are permitted, whereas previously the rules indicated that only written complaints are allowed. This change is consistent with OSHA procedural requirements under other whistleblower statutes. If a complaint is made orally, OSHA will create a written record of the complaint. Moreover, complaints may be filed in any language if the complainant is unable to file in English, and others may file on the behalf of the employee if the employee has given consent. Finally, the complainant may provide notice of withdrawal of a complaint orally or in writing.

OSHA notes that allowing oral complaints is consistent with Administrative Review Board (ARB) decisions that have long allowed oral complaints under certain environmental and asbestos statutes. Also influencing OSHA's decision is the Supreme Court's ruling in *Kasten v. Saint-Gobain Performance Plastics Corp.,* 131 S. Ct. 1325 (2011), which held that oral complaints of regulatory violations are protected under the anti-retaliation provision of the Fair Labor Standards Act. SOX does not prescribe any particular form for complaints filed under the statute.

Dodd-Frank Amendments right to review in federal court

Another change to Sarbanes-Oxley made by Dodd-Frank and reflected in the rule changes relates to the right to a jury trial in actions brought under the Sarbanes' "kickout" provision. 18 U.S.C. § 1514A (b)(1)(B). This provision gives the complainant a right to bring a *de novo* action in federal district court, regardless of the amount in controversy, if the Secretary of Labor fails to issue a final decision within 180 days of a complaint being filed, provided that the delay is not the result of bad faith on the part of the complainant.

More thorough review of parties' positions during investigation

The interim rules section pertaining to the investigation of complaints brings investigative procedures under SOX in line with procedures under other OSHA whistleblower statutes. The new rules require that during the investigatory process OSHA provide the complainant with a copy of the responding party's submission so that the complainant has an opportunity to respond. According to OSHA, this change will enhance its ability to conduct full and fair investigations and allow more thorough assessments of the respondents' defenses.

Broader relief available for whistleblowers

The new rules omit the provision in SOX which deemed reinstatement inappropriate where the respondent demonstrates that the complainant is a security risk. OSHA's explains in the interim rules that the issue of whether reinstatement is appropriate should be made "on the basis of the facts of each case and the relevant case law;" therefore, it is unnecessary to define the precise situations in which reinstatement is inappropriate. The rules also state that OSHA may order "economic reinstatement," which is similar to an order of "front pay" under the Federal Mine Safety and Health Act of 1977 and may be granted instead of the typical preliminary reinstatement when reinstatement may not be appropriate or inadvisable. Economic reinstatement requires that the employer pay the employee wages without the employee having to return to work. Employers are not entitled to choose economic reinstatement, nor do they have any basis for recovering the costs of economic reinstatement in the event that the employer eventually prevails in the adjudication.

Non-substantive changes in terminology

OSHA has made certain non-substantive changes to terminology to ensure consistency with procedural rules under other statutes. Specifically, cases under the whistleblower provision of Sarbanes-Oxley are now referred to as actions alleging "retaliation" and no longer "discrimination," individuals previously referred to in such complaints as "named persons" are now called "respondents," and "unfavorable personnel actions" are now called "adverse actions".

Interested parties are invited to comment by January 3, 2012. Comments may be submitted electronically at http://www.regulations.gov.

My problem with these rules is that it does not take into account the number of toxic tort cases that are not learned about for years after the fact. When I reported safety violation issues which exposed us to heavy metals on lead soldering, they said it was too long ago and they had no way to investigate it. I think the word of the employees that did the job should be enough. No employee is going to complain of a safety violation if they don't know there has been one and they haven't seen a material safety data sheet that would alert them to that fact!

We need to ask that these provisions take into account that the Supreme Court Law says a persons time to sue does not start until he or she learns something the company did exposed them to a toxic substance. This can be found out years after the exposure occurred and the law on reporting and compensation should include this in such cases, which the Supreme Court Law does in Ohio. This law is ineffective if ignored by the bureau of worker's comp or industrial commissions.

Write your senators and ask that the Labor Laws be honored everywhere! We also need to ask that these cases be honored according to the Supreme Court rule that states your time to sue does not start until you learn that something the company you worked for did exposed you to a toxic substance. Signing off other cases should not pre-empt this rule of law. My lawyers said they argued this fact but it was ignored. It would have helped if they had acknowledged that I said the soldering material could be absorbed through the skin.

We also need reform in Toxic Tort which would include not requiring a person to have an expert witness when the affects of exposures to chemicals and metals is backed by science supported by OSHA and the Agency for Toxic Disease Registry. This is putting too large a burden on the injured worker to prove their case. Experts are expensive as are lawyers. Workers comp was set up to be fair and impartial; I think their record speaks volumes that this has not been the case. They know someone who is disabled does not have the funds to fight a long litigious lawsuit. This is why people are losing their rights! This has to change!

This is not required for veterans exposed to Agent Orange. Their cases are allowed when there is even a casual correlation with exposure and any disease process. The government should be going after safety violators and harassers; this should not be on the shoulders of the injured workers as it has been recently. Isn't that why they set up worker's comp in the first place? No injured worker should be required to sue in civil court after they have proven their source of exposure was caused by the employer's wrongful act. They should not be required to prove the company acted with "intent to harm" as has been the case in Ohio. I was told you have to prove the company intended to cause you harm by a couple lawyers. I was also told you couldn't sue your employer. This is not what the Supreme Court Law intended when they ruled on toxic tort laws. No one can prove someone else acted with intent in my opinion. I was told I didn't have a case by one lawyer. There are laws governing employers that ignore the material safety data sheet or don't provide this information to their employees.

Case Law Regarding Toxic Torts—Ohio

"To decide weather the employer had knowledge that such a condition or procedure was dangerous, a court must examine whether the employer actually knew of the dangerous condition." "See Dailey, 138 Ohio App.3d at 582, citing Fultz v. Baja Boats, Inc. (Feb. 18, 1994), Crawford App. No. 3-93-10, 1994 Ohio App. LEXIS 623; Dailey, 138 Ohio App. 3d at 582; see also Brunn v Valley Tool & Die (Nov. 9, 1995), Cuyahoga App. No. 68811, 1995 Ohio App. Lexis 4992, Youngbird v. Whirlpool Corp. (1994), 99 Ohio App.3d 740, 746. In the context of toxic torts, such knowledge may be derived from prior accidents or the labels, warnings and material safety data sheets (MSDS) provided by the manufacturer." 2004 Gallagher, Sharp, Fulton & Norman

If you are working on any job which might expose you to a toxic substance, you should ask for the material safety data guidelines from the manufacturer of the chemical or product. Don't depend on your employer to give it to you.

I hope this book has been eye opening and has provided some much needed information to those who have been dealing with the disorders of chronic fatigue/fibromyalgia as well as any other disease process with which you might be dealing. There is some very important and eye opening research coming from Europoe and Israel. Always keep educating yourself and keep fighting the good fight. Your life and your health are too important to take for granted.

CONCLUSIONS

To make this book more user friendly, I decided to put together a guide for those newly diagnosed with CF/FM. Here is a list of tests I feel are in the order of importance when dealing with FM:

1) A comprehensive digestive stool analysis to be sure you're not dealing with any unwanted visitors to the intestinal tract and look at digestive capacity.

2) An Elisa assay that looks for immune reactions to proteins like gluten, casein etc.

3) A heavy metal challenge if you have been exposed to metals or have the symptoms of heavy metal toxicity; also liver detoxify pathways should be tested.

4) A bio 101 to find out if you are absorbing nutrients or if you are deficient in certain nutrients. Also will indicate oxidative stress on mitochondria.

5) A test to learn the status of your glutathione levels. If these are low you may not be detoxing metals and your methylation system may not be working properly.

6) Test for pyrroles if toxic. Lead can interfere with synthesis of blood production. Pyrroles form due to severe oxidative stress. I learned this from Dr. Gary Gordon's video on heavy metals.

7) Test the B-12 levels.

8) Test the function of the thyroid and adrenals.

9) Test for an imbalance in the neurotransmitters.

The one thing that has been a life saver for me has been raising the glutathione levels with the Max International Cellgevity product. I feel it is essential to give the cells the nutrition they need to detox and build the glutathione; you can do this with the Max International Cellgevity product.

Go to this site to order Cellgevity: http://www.max.com/359989

BIOGRAPHY

I live in Fishers Indiana with my husband Kent. We have been married 20 years. We moved here to be close to family. Unfortunately my son's job took him and his family to North Carolina so we are here by ourselves for now.

I started writing a blog a year ago March because I knew many people needed the information I had gathered over the last 17 years of dealing with fibromyalgia/chronic fatigue. I have had a very positive response from writing this blog and several people asked if it could be downloaded anywhere. I thought it might be helpful to put what I have learned into book form so people could reference the information and share it with others.

I have been fortunate to have found good physicians here who have been open to me sharing my research with them. They have been very concerned with trying to help me regain my health and that is truly heart warming after the experience I had in the first few years of dealing with this disorder. It is unfortunate I didn't have a lot of this knowledge in the beginning of my illness; that is why I am sharing this with you in hopes it will help guide you in the right direction.

I recommend that anyone who has been diagnosed seek a physician who has taken the time to educate himself about integrative and alternative medicine. I love Dr. Oz because he is doing his best to help people avoid the pitfalls of overly prescribed drugs and to lean on God's natural pharmacy whenever possible.

I never liked taking drugs and took them extremely sparingly when I became injured and then developed FM. Even though I was causious, I know that some of my problems no doubt came from taking some of these drugs like anti-inflammatories, cortisone, pain meds, and muscle relaxers along with my metal exposures. My tests confirm everything I have written about and everything the doctors say causes these conditions coincides with my test results.

Doctors have become more aware of the side affects of these drugs in the last few years. I have learned that there are some people whose systems are better at detoxing than others. With all the toxins in our environment, I believe our detox systems are having a hard time keeping up with all the exposures we have today. It is especially bad when you have had a direct exposure which compounds the problem.

Our genes are rapidly mutating but I wonder if they are doing this in a good way. Who knows what the environmental impact is having on those genes. I think the explosion of neurological diseases and autism are a reflection of these exposures. We need to press our legislators to recognize that we need better protections from these toxins weather it is in the workplace or in the general environment.

By sharing the research I have found over the years, I hope that it will encourage others to speak out about what has been going on and help get the changes made that will be necessary for us to survive as a country and as members of a world of nations. You need to check your nutritional status and methylation system, along with raising the glutathione before you try to chelate metals; otherwise you may be worse off then before you started. The research is showing that low glutathione levels are involved with at least 74 diseases and I believe their will be many more identified.

Researchers have indicated that metals bind up the enzymes that carry nutrition to the cells. Mercury exposure has also been linked to low glutathione levels. Raising the glutathione levels may be key in reversing any disease process. Addressing the leaky gut syndrome may also be crucial in regaining your health. Dr. Gary Gordon said in a recent video that we are all dealing with leaky gut to some degree today.

I hope I have given you some direction in restoring your health. No one should have to deal with being improperly diagnosed with the knowledge there is in research today.

RESOURCES

AFPA Articles and Newsletters "Altered Immunity and Leaky Gut Syndrome"

Annals of Allergy, Asthma and Immunology found in CFS patients

American Family Physicians "Occupational Lead Poisoning"

B.Windham (Ed.) 2009 CF/FM Scleroderma Lupus Ra MCS The Mercury Connection

Balch, Phyllis A. Prescription for Nutritional Healing, 4th ed. Penguin Group

Baylock, Russell Health and Nutrition Secrets Health Press 2006

Bell Co. research—lead soldering "Vapors generated at any pressure can be inhaled"

CDC Medical Mgt. Guidelines for Lead—Exposed Adults 4/24/07 "Urgent need to revise"

Occupational standards for lead exposure—OSHA

Cheney, Paul M.D. "The 3 R Program"

Chemical Sensitivities in Patients with FM Samual K Yue M.D. Clinical Med. Dir. Health

Chronic Neuroimmune Diseases "Common Sources of Ethyl mercury"

Doctor's Guide to Natural Medicine FM "Nutrient Deficiencies"

Dubner, Ron Ph.D. of Univ. of Maryland in Baltimore "pain that persists for hours every day leads to changes in the central nervous system."

East Pain Clinic "disautonomia"

Employment Law Book—Library ADAA Rules

EPA—Antimony and Antimony Compounds

Forester, Jonathan M.D. Conquering CFS

Fibromyalgia Network Newsletters

"Biochemical Markers Apr. '93 P. 12

Enzyme Found In Joint imbalances resulting from FMS
Kim Bennett Ph.D. 1997 July

Immune System abnormalities in CFS

Low Growth Hormone CF/FM April '93 P/13

Neurological Connections Apr. 93 P.7

Stacking The Deck On Invisible Disability Jan '92

Genova Diagnostics—Caffeine Liver Challenge Test

Genova Diagnositcs—Genetic Methylation Pathway
Testing

Genova Diagnositcs Methylation Pathway Test

Gordon Edlin Ph.D. CDC—Conditions that trigger
CFS—Other transient traumatic conditions, stress,
and toxins

Hazard Evaluation and Technical Assistance Report No.
93-0455 Page 9

Klinghart D. "Heavy Metals and Chronic Diseases" J
Explore! Article accepted for publication l/00

Live Blood Cell Analysis—"Whole Live Blood Under a
Microscope" My Blood Test

Malcome Hooper Paper, May 2001 on CF/FM

"Mastering Leptin: by Byron J. Richards, CCN with Mary
Guignon Richards

"Metabolic Origin" http://www.nutrimed.com/FIBRO.
HTM

Methylation Profile Genetic Profile Dr. Amy Yasko Genova
Diagnostics Lab

NIOSH National Institute for Occupational Safety and Health

OSHA Heavy Metals "Occupational Safety and Health Admin. Accessed online

Pub Med:
Lead (Pbo) and effect of Skin Cleansers
Low Level Environmental Lead Exposure A Continuing Challenge
Trends in Lead Exposure in Workplace and Environment

Rigden, Scott M.D. named researcher of year for CF/FM research

Rona, Zoltan P. "Leaky Gut" http://www.life-enthusiast.com/index/Articles/Rona/Leaky-Gut/l

Solder Wikipedia encyclopedia

The Arthritis Research Institute mycoplasma testing

The Basic Science of Poisons "Kloasyen CD, ed 1996 Casarett and Dovll Toxicology

The Doctor's Medical Library "Exogenous Toxins" Metals Stop Function of Enzymes" by Ron Kennedy, M.D.

The FM Syndrome Political Case Statement FM Network Kristin Thorson

"The Invisible Illnesses known as FM/CF Myofacial Pain Syndrome, Arthritis, and

Digestive Disorders Gloria Gilbere N.D., D.A. Hom., Ph. D. "Leaky Gut Syndrome"

U.S. Department of Labor /CP Analysis of Metal/Metalloid Particulates from Solder Operations

Van Koynenburg, Richard A. Ph. D. "Suggestions for Treatment of CF based on Glutathione Depletion—Methylation Cycle Block Hypothesis for the Pathogenesis of CFS

What does Your Blood Lead Level Mean? http:///www.health.state.nv.us/publications/2543
Wiley Online Library "Parental occupational lead exposure and lead concentration of newborn cord blood?